T0259389

Anemia in Older Adults

Editor

WILLIAM B. ERSHLER

CLINICS IN GERIATRIC MEDICINE

www.geriatric.theclinics.com

August 2019 • Volume 35 • Number 3

ELSEVIER

1600 John F. Kennedy Boulevard ● Suite 1800 ● Philadelphia, Pennsylvania, 19103-2899

http://www.theclinics.com

CLINICS IN GERIATRIC MEDICINE Volume 35, Number 3
August 2019 ISSN 0749–0690, ISBN-13: 978-0-323-67888-9

Editor: Jessica McCool
Developmental Editor: Laura Fisher

Clinics in Geriatric Medicine (ISSN 0749-0690) is published quarterly by Elsevier Inc., 360 Park Avenue South, New York, NY 10010-1710. Months of issue are February, May, August, and November. Business and Editorial Offices: 1600 John F. Kennedy Blvd., Suite 1800, Philadelphia, PA 191023-2899. Periodicals postage paid at New York, NY, and additional mailing offices. Subscription prices are $286.00 per year (US individuals), $632.00 per year (US institutions), $100.00 per year (US student/resident), $320.00 per year (Canadian individuals), $801.00 per year (Canadian institutions), $195.00 per year (Canadian student/resident), $402.00 per year (international individuals), $801.00 per year (international institutions), and $195.00 per year (international student/resident). Foreign air speed delivery is included in all *Clinics* subscription prices. All prices are subject to change without notice. POSTMASTER: Send address changes to *Clinics in Geriatric Medicine,* Elsevier Health Sciences Division, Subscription Customer Service, 3251 Riverport Lane, Maryland Heights, MO 63043. **Telephone: 1-800-654-2452 (U.S. and Canada); 314-447-8871 (outside U.S. and Canada). Fax: 314-447-8029. E-mail:** journalscustomerservice-usa@elsevier. com **(for print support) or** journalsonlinesupport-usa@elsevier.com **(for online support).**

Reprints. For copies of 100 or more, of articles in this publication, please contact the Commercial Reprints Department, Elsevier Inc., 360 Park Avenue South, New York, New York 10010-1710. Tel.: 212-633-3874; Fax: 212-633-3820, E-mail: reprints@elsevier.com.

Clinics in Geriatric Medicine is covered in *MEDLINE/PubMed (Index Medicus), EMBASE/Excerpta Medica, Current Contents/Clinical Medicine (CC/CM),* and the *Cumulative Index to Nursing & Allied Health Literature.*

Contributors

EDITOR

WILLIAM B. ERSHLER, MD
Director, Division of Benign Hematology, Inova Schar Cancer Institute, Inova Fairfax Hospital, Falls Church, Virginia, USA

AUTHORS

HAIRIL RIZAL ABDULLAH, MMed (Anaesthesiology)
Senior Consultant, Department of Anaesthesiology, Singapore General Hospital, Singapore, Singapore

SYED ASHAD ABID, MD, MPH
Fellow, Geriatric Medicine, Division of Geriatrics and Palliative Care, Department of Medicine, Rhode Island Hospital, The Warren Alpert Medical School of Brown University, Providence, Rhode Island, USA

MICHAEL AUERBACH, MD, FACP
Auerbach Hematology and Oncology, Baltimore, Maryland, USA; Clinical Professor of Medicine, Georgetown University School of Medicine, Washington, DC, USA

JOSEPH L. BLACKSHEAR, MD
Professor of Medicine, Consultant, Department of Cardiovascular Diseases, Mayo Clinic, Jacksonville, Florida, USA

WILLIAM B. ERSHLER, MD
Director, Division of Benign Hematology, Inova Schar Cancer Institute, Inova Fairfax Hospital, Falls Church, Virginia, USA

STEFAN GRAVENSTEIN, MD, MPH
Division of Geriatrics and Palliative Care, Professor, Department of Medicine, Rhode Island Hospital, The Warren Alpert Medical School of Brown University, Department of Health Services Policy and Practice, School of Public Health, Providence Veterans Administration Medical Center, Brown University, Providence, Rhode Island, USA

EMMA M. GROARKE, MD
Fellow, Hematology Branch, National Heart, Lung, and Blood Institute, National Institutes of Health, Mark Hatfield Clinical Research Center, Bethesda, Maryland, USA

SEAN X. LENG, MD, PhD
Professor, Department of Medicine, Division of Geriatric Medicine and Gerontology, Johns Hopkins School of Medicine, Baltimore, Maryland, USA

FRANCO MUSIO, MD
Associate Professor, Department of Medicine, Inova Fairfax Hospital, Virginia Commonwealth University School of Medicine, Annandale, Virginia, USA; Nephrology Associates of Northern Virginia, Fairfax, Virginia, USA

AMAN NANDA, MD
Division of Geriatrics and Palliative Care, Associate Professor, Department of Medicine, Rhode Island Hospital, The Warren Alpert Medical School of Brown University, Providence, Rhode Island, USA

ARUN S. SHET, MD, PhD
Sickle Cell Branch, National Heart Lung and Blood Institute, National Institutes of Health, Bethesda, Maryland, USA

YILIN EILEEN SIM, MMed (Anaesthesiology)
Associate Consultant, Department of Anaesthesiology, Singapore General Hospital, Singapore, Singapore

JERRY SPIVAK, MD
Professor of Medicine, Johns Hopkins School of Medicine, Baltimore, Maryland, USA

JULIETTE TAVENIER, MSc
PhD Student, Clinical Research Centre, Copenhagen University Hospital Hvidovre, Hvidovre, Denmark

SWEE LAY THEIN, MBBS, DSc
Senior Investigator and Chief, Sickle Cell Branch, National Heart Lung and Blood Institute, National Institutes of Health, Bethesda, Maryland, USA

NEAL S. YOUNG, MD
Senior Investigator, Hematology Branch, National Heart, Lung, and Blood Institute, National Institutes of Health, Mark Hatfield Clinical Research Center, Bethesda, Maryland, USA

CHAD ZIK, MD
Assistant Professor of Internal Medicine, Virginia Commonwealth University School of Medicine Inova Campus, Fairfax, Virginia, USA

Contents

Video content accompanies this article at http://www.geriatric.
theclinics.com.

Heyde described aortic stenosis and gastrointestinal bleeding in the 1950s. Since then, a link with intestinal angiodysplasia and abnormalities of von Willebrand factor (VWF) has been noted. Loss of the highest-molecular-weight multimers of VWF and bleeding also have been described in subaortic stenosis in hypertrophic cardiomyopathy, in isolated mitral and aortic insufficiency, in endocarditis, in patients with prosthetic valve stenosis or regurgitation, and in patients with left ventricular assist devices (LVADs). Bleeding tends to recur with local treatment of angiodysplasias, whereas cardiac repair or removal of LVAD eliminates VWF dysfunction is curative of bleeding in the majority.

Anemia has a higher prevalence among residents of long-term care setting. Signs and symptoms of anemia in this group are more insidious and can be overlooked and attributed to other disease manifestations or old age. Available data on the consequences of anemia suggest worse outcomes in heart failure; cognitive and functional decline; and increased rates of falls, hospitalizations, and mortality. Diagnosis and treatment of anemia in long-term care residents should be considered based on cost and benefit to the patient and patient's and/or caregiver's preferences.

Anemia in the elderly is common and is associated with exposure to blood transfusion and higher perioperative morbidity and mortality. These patients would benefit from early diagnosis and work-up of the cause of pre-operative anemia systematically. This can be done in preoperative anemia clinics as part of an overall patient blood management program. Iron-deficiency anemia is amenable to treatment with oral or intravenous iron. Intravenous iron leads to a more rapid hemoglobin response, and is devoid of gastrointestinal side effects. More data are needed to determine if pre-operative correction of iron-deficiency anemia reduces the morbidity associated with anemia.

CLINICS IN GERIATRIC MEDICINE

SERIES OF RELATED INTEREST

Hematology/Oncology Clinics
Medical Clinics of North America
Primary Care: Clinics in Office Practice

THE CLINICS ARE AVAILABLE ONLINE!
Access your subscription at:
www.theclinics.com

Preface

Anemia in the Elderly: Not to be Ignored

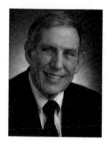

William B. Ershler, MD
Editor

Readers of *Clinics in Geriatric Medicine* are well aware of the demographic shifts throughout all world populations—industrialized or not—resulting in constantly increasing numbers of old and very-old individuals. Some of this is based upon increased birth rates after the Second World War, but also longer survival resulting from healthier life style and reduction in early deaths from acute illnesses including infection, coronary artery disease and cancer. As a consequence, chronic diseases such as diabetes, atherosclerotic vascular disease, arthritis and Alzheimer's have become more prevalent, as has the numbers of patients with two or more of these chronic illnesses (comorbidities).

It has been a long-held notion that anemia is not part of normal aging and any increased prevalence with advancing age is the result of coexisting disease(s). Yet, even with normal aging there is a decline in hemoglobin level, but typically to levels that remain within the normal range. Nonetheless, epidemiologic studies have demonstrated that approximately 11% of community-dwelling individuals over the age of 65 years have anemia—most likely reflecting the existence of chronic illness in this age group. In fact, the percent with anemia increases with each decade beyond 50 and reaches levels in excess of 50% in individuals who meet criteria for frailty.

What is critically important is that even mild anemia is associated with a panoply of adverse consequences that include impaired physical function, cognition and quality of life—not to mention need for hospitalization, surgical complications, length of hospital stay, need for long-term care after hospital discharge, and increased mortality.

It is easy for clinicians to make a diagnosis of anemia. However, in older patients with mild anemia, unless secondary to iron or B12 deficiency, it remains unclear how far to pursue the mechanism, whether or not it should be treated, and if so, how. There is very little existing evidence on which to base these important decisions. In truth, what we have is a dearth of data and a wide open domain for active clinical research.

Clin Geriatr Med 35 (2019) ix–x
https://doi.org/10.1016/j.cger.2019.05.001
0749-0690/19/© 2019 Elsevier Inc. All rights reserved.

In this issue of *Clinics in Geriatric Medicine* there are contributions that will serve as reviews and updates of the common causes of anemia in the elderly (iron and B12 deficiency, renal insufficiency and inflammation), perioperative implications and a discussion of what is increasingly recognized as "unexplained anemia of the elderly" or UAE. Two additional comprehensive reports from the NIH have been included: one a basic review of aging and hematopoiesis and the second on sickle cell anemia in older adults. An additional intriguing report features Heyde's syndrome, with resulting anemia that is very likely more prevalent in older people with aortic valve disease or other cardiac conditions than is currently appreciated.

We anticipate this issue will be of value to clinicians serving in the broad field of geriatric medicine and will also serve investigators to generate new hypotheses for basic or clinical research. There are a lot of questions that remain to be answered. For example, although the associations of anemia and adverse outcomes are clearly delineated, it remains to be established whether correcting mild to moderate anemia, particularly for the significant portion with "unexplained" anemia, will result in improvements in these outcomes. The "geriatric imperative" is upon us now and we really should not ignore the importance of anemia.

William B. Ershler, MD
Director, Benign Hematology Division
Inova Schar Cancer Institute
Inova Fairfax Medical Center
3300 Gallows Road, Suite O-581
Falls Church, VA 22042, USA

E-mail address:
william.ershler@inova.org

Aging and Hematopoiesis

Emma M. Groarke, MD*, Neal S. Young, MD

KEYWORDS

- Hematopoiesis • Anemia in the elderly
- Clonal hematopoiesis of indeterminate potential
- Clonal cytopenia of undetermined significance

KEY POINTS

- With age, both the overall number of stem cells and the rate of cell division increase, but functionally these hematopoietic stem cells seem inferior.
- A decrease in lymphoid progenitors contributes to lymphopenia and likely to decreased immunity in the elderly.
- Clonal hematopoiesis of indeterminate potential (CHIP) is defined as the presence of a somatic mutation associated with hematological malignancy in the absence of a cytopenia.
- CHIP is common in the elderly and has been associated with an increased risk of both hematological malignancy and atherosclerosis.
- Clonal cytopenia of undetermined significance (CCUS) is defined as cytopenias associated with a myeloid somatic mutation but not meeting the criteria for myelodysplastic syndrome. CCUS has a significant rate of progression to myeloid neoplasm.

INTRODUCTION

As humans age, many changes take place in the bone marrow, which may have clinical consequences. Differences in the marrow between young and old have been demonstrated in both animal models and in humans, involving alterations in overall cell number, senescence, lineage differentiation, cellular composition, and function of the hematopoietic stem cell (HSC). These changes likely contribute to a higher rate of cytopenias, predominantly anemia and lymphopenia, and a risk of hematological malignancy.

As stem cells reproduce, they naturally acquire mutations that are then passed on to their progeny—producing a clonal hematopoiesis. Acquired mutations found in HSCs are not necessarily pathogenic and they normally and inevitably accumulate over time.[1] Clonal hematopoiesis of indeterminate potential (CHIP) is described as the

Disclosure Statement: The authors have nothing to disclose.
Hematology Branch, National Heart, Lung, and Blood Institute, National Institutes of Health, Mark Hatfield Clinical Research Center, Room 3E-5140, 10 Center Drive, Bethesda, MD 20891-1202, USA
* Corresponding author.
E-mail address: emma.groarke@nih.gov

presence of known somatic mutations in genes long associated with myeloid hematological disorders and is common in the normal aging population. It remains unclear whether clonal hematopoiesis is a disease or an accompaniment of normal aging. In retrospective population studies, CHIP has been shown associated with the development of both hematological malignancy (lymphoid and myeloid) and atherosclerosis (cardiovascular and cerebrovascular disease).[2]

ALTERED BLOOD COUNTS WITH AGING

Anemia in the elderly is prevalent, in 11% of men and 10% of women 65 years and older, and it is multifactorial.[3] Common etiologies include anemia of chronic disease associated with inflammation, chronic kidney disease, nutritional deficiencies (such as iron, vitamin B_{12}, and folate deficiencies), and clonal disorders, such as myelodysplastic syndrome (MDS). These topics are covered elsewhere in this issue.

There has been no specific decrease in the erythroid population noted when evaluating marrow function. Levels of erythropoietin (EPO), a hormone that stimulates erythropoiesis, are increased. It is possible that, as humans age, their response to EPO stimulation is decreased and higher levels are required to maintain a normal hemoglobin level. Patients with inflammatory disorders have lower blood concentrations of EPO, suggesting less hormonal stimulation as an explanation for anemia in this circumstance.[4]

An elevated white blood cell count is an independent marker of all-cause mortality,[5] specifically correlating with cancer or cardiovascular-related death,[6] in all populations, including the elderly. Leukocytosis may reflect generalized inflammation.

Monocytes increase with age. In murine models, monocytes from aged mice promote intimal hyperplasia, a feature of atherosclerosis, compared with monocytes from young mice. In addition, up-regulation of genes involved in cellular adhesion and inflammation is a feature of aged monocytes.[7] In humans, alterations occur in the phenotype and cell surface markers of monocytes from classical $CD14^+CD16^-$ to nonclassical $CD14^+CD16^+$, with an increase in nonclassical monocytes seen with age. Nonclassical monocytes secrete proinflammatory cytokines[8] but with unknown consequences.

PHYSIOLOGY AND PATHOPHYSIOLOGY OF STEM CELL AGING

Hematopoiesis is the continuous process by which blood cells are produced, maintained at normal levels, and increased in response to demand. HSCs have 3 critical properties: differentiation into progenitors of all lineages; high proliferative capacity, as a progenitor giving rise to many thousands of mature blood cells; and self-renewal to maintain the HSC pool. The major point where lineages diverge is between 2 common progenitors—myeloid and lymphoid. The primitive myeloid progenitor is responsible for the production of granulocytes, erythroid cells (red cell precursors), and megakaryocytes (platelet precursors) and the lymphoid progenitor for the production of lymphocytes. The marrow stroma, vasculature, and cytokines of the marrow environment play a role in stem cell biology.[9]

Mouse Models

In young mice, HSC cell turnover is infrequent, approximately 1 division every 30 days. In comparing young and old mice, there is a 2-fold increase of HSCs in the older mouse, measured by competitive repopulation. In the competitive repopulation assay, marrow cells from young and old mice are mixed, and these cell mixtures are transplanted to repopulate irradiated recipients. Skewing, or increased numbers, of myeloid progenitor cells compared with lymphoid progenitor cells also has been observed in mice using transplantation of younger and older mouse bone marrow and ascertaining myeloid and lymphoid chimerism.[10] Telomere shortening, which occurs with age, may play a role in myeloid skewing by activation of interferon gamma, thus inducing an inflammatory response.[11]

Numbers and Senescence

Human stem cells are difficult to study. Immunophenotyping identifies HSCs by specific cell surface markers using antibodies. Standard immunotyping is fluorescence based, and there are limits to the number of cell surface markers that can be identified on a single cell. Additionally, sample quality (especially dilution with peripheral blood) and sampling site may affect results.

In humans, as with mice, the bone marrow seems to have increased numbers of multipotent stem cells with increased age, by immunophenotype, despite its hypocellular morphologic appearance. Aged HSCs have a higher rate of cell division and proliferation (active phases of the cell cycle) than do younger stem cells, which tend to be quiescent (inactive phase of the cell cycle).[12]

Lineage

As cells age, they show up-regulation in genes associated with growth and proliferation as well as those associated with myeloid malignancies.[13] By immunophenotyping of lymphoid and myeloid cell markers in humans, there is a preservation of numbers of myeloid cells and a decrease in B-lymphoid cells, skewing the myeloid-to-lymphoid ratio and resulting in myeloid predominance,[12,14] an effect also seen in mice. Skewing may explain the greater increased prevalence of myeloid compared with lymphoid malignancies apparent with age.[15]

The reduction in cells differentiated to the B-lymphoid lineage, combined with an overall reduction in T-cell production,[16] may explain the lymphopenia associated with aging and contribute to impaired immunity in the elderly.

Cellular Factors

Many cellular factors have been shown to contribute to HSC aging: molecular signaling pathways, such as those involved in DNA repair; changes in mitochondrial function, causing reduced enzymatic activity and the acquisition of somatic mutations; reduction in cell polarity, resulting in altered cell division; and shortening of telomeres.[17–20]

Function

Although HSC numbers increase with age, their functionality may be impaired. Oxidative DNA damage may hinder self-replication.[12] In HSC transplants, older age of the donor associates with decreased overall survival,[21–23] and, with autologous stem cell transplants, older patients have poorer engraftment.[24] In addition, stem cells from older donor animals have reduced engraftment compared with those from younger mice.

AGING CLONES

Defining clonality is difficult. Classically, in the field of hematology-oncology, clones are described as a uniform population of malignant cells. Malignant clones evolve, acquiring further subclones, and ultimately may cause disease. Clonality also applies, however, to normal hematopoiesis. As cells divide, they, by definition, produce a clone of themselves. During this process cell alterations may occur, including mutations, which may be either pathogenic or nonpathogenic.

Because HSCs must undergo multiple divisions to sustain hematopoiesis, they are susceptible, over time, to accumulate mutations, which are inherited by their descendant cells. Mutations also occur due to environmental factors, such as chemicals and radiation. The average person acquires 10 to 20 nonpathogenic passenger mutations per stem cell by middle age.[1] Mutations likely confer a survival advantage over nonmutated stem cells, resulting in proliferation of a clonal population or clonal hematopoiesis. Skewed X chromosome inactivation, particularly in older patients, was an early if nonspecific indication of this phenomenon.[25]

Clonal hematopoiesis has been detected using a barcode method—measuring for the presence of somatic mutations without a specific driver gene. In 1 large study looking at an Icelandic population, the presence of clonal hematopoiesis increased from 0.5% in those less than 35 years to more than 50% for subjects older than 85 years.[26] Clonal hematopoiesis was associated with a reduction in overall survival, a finding that likely reflects a degree of overall cell damage.

The population size and lifetime dynamics of HSCs were recently investigated by measuring naturally occurring somatic mutations in a single individual (with normal blood counts and no evidence of hematological disease) and imputing an evolutionary tree. The subject had no mutations associated with myeloid malignancy (CHIP). By computation, there seemed to be hundreds of thousands of stem cells at any 1 time, a much higher figure than previously estimated, with cell division at intervals of 2 months to 20 months. There was a close ancestral relationship between differentiated granulocytes and differentiated B lymphocytes but not between granulocytes and T lymphocytes, suggesting divergence in ancestry.

THE DEFINITION AND PATHOPHYSIOLOGY CLONAL HEMATOPOIESIS OF INDETERMINATE POTENTIAL

CHIP is a form of clonal hematopoiesis where a somatic driver mutation associated with hematological malignancy is present without morphologic evidence of bone marrow dysplasia or neoplasia.[27] A clone size, or variant allele fraction (VAF), of at least 2% has been used in the literature as a defined cutoff, although smaller clones can be detected using deeper sequencing techniques. Such mutations occur in leukocytes and have been found in a substantial proportion of the healthy aging population by next-generation sequencing. CHIP may represent a preneoplastic phase of hematological malignancy, in particular myeloid disorders, but also is associated with lymphoid malignancy and plasma cell dyscrasias.[28–31] Most people with these mutations do not develop a hematological malignancy, with a risk of progression of 0.5% to 1% per year.[32]

There are several specific myeloid genes associated with CHIP, the most common being *DNMT3A*, *TET2*, and *ASXL1*, and some spliceosome mutations. CHIP mutations preferentially affect the myeloid lineage and natural killer cells based on a higher VAF than seen that in B cells and T cells of the same sample.[33]

CLONAL HEMATOPOIESIS OF INDETERMINATE POTENTIAL AND HEMATOLOGICAL DISORDERS

Few patients with CHIP actually develop myeloid neoplasms despite the association.[27] It is estimated that its presence doubles the risk of developing a hematological malignancy—however, these are not common malignancies, with MDS having an incidence of 0.22 per 100,000 to 13.2 per 100,000 and acute myeloid leukemia (AML) having an incidence of 0.6 to 11 per 100,000, combining all ages, genders, and risk factors.[34]

CHIP has been associated with all types of hematological malignancy, including MDS, AML, chronic lymphocytic leukemia, acute lymphoblastic leukemia/lymphoma, myeloproliferative neoplasms, lymphoma, and myeloma, although in studies the overall numbers of patients who developed hematological malignancy is low.[32] The presence of greater than 1 somatic mutation and increased VAF positively predict for malignant progression. Certain mutations (such as *IDH* and spliceosome mutations) are correlated more strongly with this progression than are the more common *DNMT3A, TET2,* and *ASXL1.* These latter mutations may represent a founder event that renders the environment more susceptible to further leukemogenesis rather than a direct neoplastic trigger.[35]

In one recent study, the presence of CHIP mutations in AML patients was sought in samples collected years prior to disease development to identify ways of predicting risk of progression to AML. The presence of a CHIP mutation (except *DNMT3A* and *TET2*) doubled the risk of developing AML per 5% increase in clone size. *DNMT3A* and *TET2* conferred a lower risk of progression than *TP53* and *U2AF1* (a spliceosome mutation) which conferred a higher risk. AML patients had significantly higher numbers of mutations and larger clones than a control group without AML. Mutations commonly seen in AML, such as *FLT3, NPM1,* and *CEBPA,* were absent in historic samples, suggesting that these occur later in leukemogenesis. Red cell distribution width (RDW) was identified as a routine clinical test that had a significant correlation to risk of progression to AML and may act as a screening tool.[30]

CHIP mutations have been observed in aplastic anemia at a rate of 47%, with *BCOR, BCORL1,* and *PIGA* the most commonly seen mutations, correlating with a better response to therapy and higher progression-free survival. *DNMT3A* and *ASXL1* also were common but were collectively associated with poorer outcomes.[36]

CLONAL HEMATOPOIESIS OF INDETERMINATE POTENTIAL AND ATHEROSCLEROSIS

CHIP has been associated with an increased atherosclerotic risk,[2,37] in particular, cardiovascular and cerebrovascular disease. Cardiovascular disease has been shown 2-fold to 4-fold higher in patients with CHIP, with an increase in both myocardial infarction and coronary artery calcification, using retrospective data. This association was significantly correlated with a higher VAF (>10%). The presence of greater than 1 somatic mutation was linked to an increased prevalence of peripheral vascular disease and diabetes[33] compared with those with 1 mutation. Both *DNMT3A* and *TET2* have been associated with worse long-term clinical outcomes in patients with congestive heart failure.[38]

Mutational loss of *TET2* has been associated with increased risk of atherosclerosis in murine models. Explanations include an inflammatory response with macrophage dysfunction causing plaque build-up or leukocytosis effect similar to that seen in myeloproliferative disorders. The loss of *TET2* increased monocytes and interleukin (IL)-6 in murine and human bone marrow.[39,40] TET2 seems to play a role in the regulation of IL-6, an inflammatory cytokine, and may be associated with a proinflammatory state and increased atherosclerotic risk. With further study, this inflammatory process may become a target of future therapeutic agents.

CLONAL CYTOPENIAS OF UNDETERMINED SIGNIFICANCE

Idiopathic cytopenia of undetermined significance (ICUS) is used to describe an unexplained cytopenia not meeting MDS diagnostic criteria that cannot be explained by

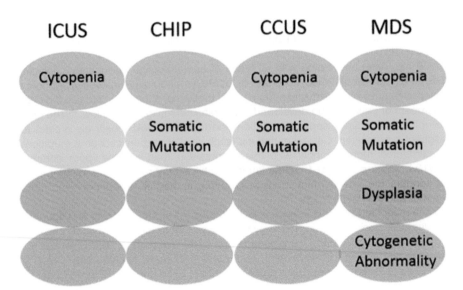

Fig. 1. Distinction between ICUS, CHIP, CCUS, and MDS.

any other hematologic or nonhematologic disease process.[41] Clinical confusion has long existed as to the optimal follow-up for these patients. Recently, it has been shown that many patients with unexplained cytopenia harbor a myeloid somatic mutation. In one study, this was true for approximately two-thirds of patients who historically had been diagnosed with ICUS.[42]

Clonal cytopenia of undetermined significance (CCUS) is defined as a cytopenia and associated myeloid somatic mutation in the absence of morphologic evidence of MDS or an MDS defining cytogenetic abnormality[43,44] (**Fig. 1**). In a study looking at patients with unexplained cytopenia (previously classed as ICUS), the presence of a myeloid somatic mutation (CCUS) significantly increased the risk of progression to a myeloid neoplasm (95% risk vs 9% risk at 10 years). Risk of progression to leukemia was similar to that of low-risk MDS. Risk factors for progression identified included the presence of spliceosome mutations, having greater than 1 mutation, and a large clone size. These data suggest that these patients should be clinically monitored as high-risk patients, similarly to patients with MDS, rather than persons with standard CHIP, who have a much lower progression risk and are likely to have a normal life span.[42] Additionally, patients with ICUS, in whom CCUS has been excluded, have a lower risk of progression than those with an identified mutation.

SUMMARY

With age, changes take place in bone marrow hematopoiesis that can have an impact on health and longevity. Overall, human stem cells seem to become more poorly functional and, possibly as a result, have an increase in both their number and cell dividing capacity. Myeloid skewing also becomes apparent with age and may contribute to the increased rates of myeloid malignancy in the elderly. This skewing, coupled with a reduction in T-cell production, results in a decrease in lymphocytes, which may contribute to a decrease in immunity seen in the elderly. Although erythroid progenitors do not seem to decrease with age, increased rates of anemia may be explained by changes in their response to EPO.

Clonal hematopoiesis is prevalent with aging and is increasingly identified with the advent of more sequencing. A majority of individuals with CHIP do not develop hematological malignancy and many of those who do develop it acquire a further driver mutation that promotes leukemogenesis. Certain higher-risk populations with CHIP have been identified—in particular those with more than 1 mutation and a higher allele burden. CCUS also is classed as higher risk with a significant rate of progression to hematological malignancy demonstrated in 1 study. The association between CHIP and atherosclerosis warrants further study, given the high incidence and prevalence of atherosclerosis in the general population, particularly in older age groups. Prospective studies further investigating clonal hematopoiesis are needed both to develop a method of risk stratification for the clinical hematologist and to identify any potential future therapeutic targets.

REFERENCES

1. Cooper JN, Young NS. Clonality in context: hematopoietic clones in their marrow environment. Blood 2017;130(22):2363–72.
2. Jaiswal S, Natarajan P, Silver AJ, et al. Clonal hematopoiesis and risk of atherosclerotic cardiovascular disease. N Engl J Med 2017;377(2):111–21.
3. Guralnik JM, Eisenstaedt RS, Ferrucci L, et al. Prevalence of anemia in persons 65 years and older in the United States: evidence for a high rate of unexplained anemia. Blood 2004;104(8):2263–8.
4. Ershler WB, Sheng S, McKelvey J, et al. Serum erythropoietin and aging: a longitudinal analysis. J Am Geriatr Soc 2005;53(8):1360–5.
5. Willems JM, Trompet S, Blauw GJ, et al. White blood cell count and C-reactive protein are independent predictors of mortality in the oldest old. J Gerontol A Biol Sci Med Sci 2010;65(7):764–8.
6. Grimm RH, Neaton JD, Ludwig W, et al. Prognostic importance of the white blood cell count for coronary, cancer, and all-cause mortality. JAMA 1985;254(14): 1932–7.
7. Martinez L, Gomez C, Vazquez-Padron R. Age-related changes in monocytes exacerbate neointimal hyperplasia after vascular injury. Oncotarget 2015;6(19): 17054–64.
8. Seidler S, Zimmermann HW, Bartneck M, et al. Age-dependent alterations of monocyte subsets and monocyte-related chemokine pathways in healthy adults. BMC Immunol 2010;11(1):30.
9. Sallman DA, Cluzeau T, Basiorka AA, et al. Unraveling the pathogenesis of MDS: the NLRP3 inflammasome and pyroptosis drive the MDS phenotype. Front Oncol 2016;6:151.
10. Sudo K, Ema H, Morita Y, et al. Age-associated characteristics of murine hematopoietic stem cells. J Exp Med 2000;192(9):1273–80.
11. Chen J, Bryant MA, Dent JJ, et al. Hematopoietic lineage skewing and intestinal epithelia degeneration in aged mice with telomerase RNA component deletion. Exp Gerontol 2015;72:251–60.
12. Pang WW, Price EA, Sahoo D, et al. Human bone marrow hematopoietic stem cells are increased in frequency and myeloid-biased with age. Proc Natl Acad Sci U S A 2011;108(50):20012–7.
13. Akunuru SG. Hartmut, aging, clonality, and Rejuvenation of hematopoietic stem cells. Trends Mol Med 2016;22(8):701–12.
14. Kuranda K, Vargaftig J, de la Rochere P, et al. Age-related changes in human hematopoietic stem/progenitor cells. Aging Cell 2011;10(3):542–6.

15. Signer RAJ, Montecino-Rodriguez E, Witte ON, et al. Age-related defects in B lymphopoiesis underlie the myeloid dominance of adult leukemia. Blood 2007; 110(6):1831–9.
16. Dorshkind K, Montecino-Rodriguez E, Signer RA. The ageing immune system: is it ever too old to become young again? Nat Rev Immunol 2009;9(1):57–62.
17. Yao YG, Ellison FM, McCoy JP, et al. Age-dependent accumulation of mtDNA mutations in murine hematopoietic stem cells is modulated by the nuclear genetic background. Hum Mol Genet 2007;16(3):286–94.
18. Van Zant G, Liang Y. Concise review: hematopoietic stem cell aging, life span, and transplantation. Stem Cells Transl Med 2012;1(9):651–7.
19. Calado RT, Dumitriu B. Telomere dynamics in mice and humans. Semin Hematol 2013;50(2):165–74.
20. Florian MC, Geiger H. Concise review: polarity in stem cells, disease, and aging. Stem Cells 2010;28(9):1623–9.
21. Kollman C, Howe CW, Anasetti C, et al. Donor characteristics as risk factors in recipients after transplantation of bone marrow from unrelated donors: the effect of donor age. Blood 2001;98(7):2043–51.
22. Kollman C, Spellman SR, Zhang MJ, et al. The effect of donor characteristics on survival after unrelated donor transplantation for hematologic malignancy. Blood 2016;127(2):260–7.
23. Finke J, Schmoor C, Bethge WA. Prognostic factors affecting outcome after allogeneic transplantation for hematological malignancies from unrelated donors: results from a randomized trial. Biol Blood Marrow Transplant 2012;18(11):1716–26.
24. Woolthuis CM, Mariani N, Verkaik-Schakel RN, et al. Aging impairs long-term hematopoietic regeneration after autologous stem cell transplantation. Biol Blood Marrow Transplant 2014;20(6):865–71.
25. Anger B, Janssen JW, Schrezenmeier H, et al. Clonal analysis of chronic myeloproliferative disorders using X-linked DNA polymorphisms. Leukemia 1990;4(4): 258–61.
26. Zink F, Stacey SN, Norddahl GL, et al. Clonal hematopoiesis, with and without candidate driver mutations, is common in the elderly. Blood 2017;130(6):742–52.
27. Steensma DP, Bejar R, Jaiswal S, et al. Clonal hematopoiesis of indeterminate potential and its distinction from myelodysplastic syndromes. Blood 2015;126(1): 9–16.
28. Jaiswal S, Fontanillas P, Flannick J, et al. Age-related clonal hematopoiesis associated with adverse outcomes. N Engl J Med 2014;371(26):2488–98.
29. Welch JS, Ley TJ, Link DC, et al. The origin and evolution of mutations in acute myeloid leukemia. Cell 2012;150(2):264–78.
30. Abelson S, Collord G, Ng SWK, et al. Prediction of acute myeloid leukaemia risk in healthy individuals. Nature 2018;559(7714):400–4.
31. Desai P, Mencia-Trinchant N, Savenkov O, et al. Somatic mutations precede acute myeloid leukemia years before diagnosis. Nat Med 2018;24(7):1015–23.
32. Genovese G, Kähler AK, Handsaker RE, et al. Clonal hematopoiesis and blood-cancer risk inferred from blood DNA sequence. N Engl J Med 2014;371(26): 2477–87.
33. Arends CM, Galan-Sousa J, Hoyer K, et al. Hematopoietic lineage distribution and evolutionary dynamics of clonal hematopoiesis. Leukemia 2018;32(9): 1908–19.
34. Lubeck DP, et al. Systematic literature review of the global incidence and prevalence of myelodysplastic syndrome and acute myeloid leukemia. Blood 2016; 128(22):5930.

35. Xie M, Lu C, Wang J, et al. Age-related mutations associated with clonal hematopoietic expansion and malignancies. Nat Med 2014;20(12):1472–8.
36. Yoshizato T, et al. Somatic mutations and clonal hematopoiesis in aplastic anemia. N Engl J Med 2015;373(1):35–47.
37. Fuster JJ, MacLauchlan S, Zuriaga MA, et al. Clonal hematopoiesis associated with TET2 deficiency accelerates atherosclerosis development in mice. Science 2017;355(6327):842–7.
38. Dorsheimer L, Assmus B, Rasper T, et al. Association of mutations contributing to clonal hematopoiesis with prognosis in chronic ischemic heart failure. JAMA Cardiol 2019;4(1):25–33.
39. Cull AH, Snetsinger B, Buckstein R, et al. Tet2 restrains inflammatory gene expression in macrophages. Exp Hematol 2017;55:56–70.e13.
40. Zhang Q, Zhao K, Shen Q, et al. Tet2 is required to resolve inflammation by recruiting Hdac2 to specifically repress IL-6. Nature 2015;525(7569):389–93.
41. Valent P, Horny HP, Bennett JM, et al. Definitions and standards in the diagnosis and treatment of the myelodysplastic syndromes: consensus statements and report from a working conference. Leuk Res 2007;31(6):727–36.
42. Malcovati L, Gallì A, Travaglino E, et al. Clinical significance of somatic mutation in unexplained blood cytopenia. Blood 2017;129(25):3371–8.
43. Cargo CA, Rowbotham N, Evans PA, et al. Targeted sequencing identifies patients with preclinical MDS at high risk of disease progression. Blood 2015; 126(21):2362–5.
44. Kwok B, Hall JM, Witte JS, et al. MDS-associated somatic mutations and clonal hematopoiesis are common in idiopathic cytopenias of undetermined significance. Blood 2015;126(21):2355–61.

Unexplained Anemia in the Elderly

William B. Ershler, MD

KEYWORDS

- Unexplained anemia • Elderly • Comorbidity

KEY POINTS

- Despite research conducted to demystify unexplained anemia in the elderly (UAE), there remains a healthy subset of anemia (30%–50%) that cannot be more confidently classified than "unexplained."
- UAE has emerged as a stand-alone clinical entity, likely representing an amalgam of age and/or disease-altered physiologies.
- Coincident with our recognition of UAE, there has developed a robust literature of primarily observational studies in which unfavorable geriatric outcomes have been linked to even mild decrements in hemoglobin level.

On examining a large data set for the prevalence and mechanisms explaining the occurrence of anemia in community-dwelling older people, Guralnik and colleagues[1] described a category that they termed "unexplained anemia of the elderly" (UAE).[2]

Hematologists, generally not modest when considering matters relating to blood, may take umbrage at the term "unexplained" and construct explanatory mechanisms for such anemia from data at hand (eg, a little bit of iron deficiency, low-level inflammation, androgen deficiency with added renal insufficiency, and possibly nascent myelodysplasia) but still, despite research conducted to demystify UAE, there remains a healthy subset of anemia (30%–50%) that cannot be more confidently classified than "unexplained." Thus, UAE has emerged as a stand-alone clinical entity, likely representing an amalgam of age and/or disease-altered physiologies.

Coincident with our recognition of UAE, there has developed a robust literature, primarily observational, in which unfavorable geriatric outcomes have been linked to even mild decrements in hemoglobin level.

CONSEQUENCES OF ANEMIA IN GERIATRIC POPULATIONS

Approximately 10% of community-dwelling older adults have anemia based on the application of the commonly used World Health Organization (WHO) thresholds of

Disclosure: The author has nothing to disclose.
Division of Benign Hematology, Inova Schar Cancer Institute, Inova Fairfax Hospital, 3300 Gallows Road, Suite O-581, Falls Church, VA 22042, USA
E-mail address: william.ershler@inova.org

Clin Geriatr Med 35 (2019) 295–305
https://doi.org/10.1016/j.cger.2019.03.002

hemoglobin <13 g/dL for men and less than 12 g/dL for women.[1,3-6] Anemia in older people, particularly unexplained anemia (UA) (as described in the section entitled DEFINING UNEXPLAINED ANEMIA below) tends to be mild, with hemoglobin levels typically 1 g/dL below the WHO standard. Yet, a large and expanding literature describes the association of anemia with distinct morbidities and mortality. For example, having anemia is associated with increased hospitalization[7-9] and longer hospital stays.[10] Low hemoglobin levels also associate with cognitive decline,[11] depression,[12] impaired quality of life,[13] diminished overall physical function,[14] falls,[15] and, as mentioned, higher mortality.[10,16,17] Considering demographic trends indicating that within 3 decades approximately 25% of the world's population will be 60 years or older,[18] the overall societal burden of anemia is, and will increasingly become, even more substantial.

Yet, there remains no definitive consensus that anemia treatment favorably affects any of these associated adverse outcomes. In this review, we expand on what is and is not known about UAE and provide a framework for when to intervene.

PHYSIOLOGIC PATHWAYS TO ANEMIA IN THE ELDERLY

Beyond 50 years of age, anemia occurs more frequently with each advancing decade, and is particularly prevalent among the most frail (**Tables 1–3**).[1,4,5,17,19-22] Approximately 10% of community-dwelling adults older than 65 have anemia based on the previously mentioned WHO thresholds for diagnosis.[1,4-6] Anemia prevalence varies significantly by race: the lower median hemoglobin in elderly African American individuals translates to a threefold higher prevalence compared with white individuals.[1,23,24] Yet, the adverse consequences of even mild anemia experienced in the general population is not observed in mildly anemic African American individuals.[25]

Strategies to uncover an etiology of anemia is essentially no different for older than younger adults. From a rather limited data set including hemoglobin level, red blood cell indices, and serum chemistries, a single cause of anemia can be defined for most cases, particularly in younger patients. For example, iron deficiency in menstruating women or renal insufficiency in a diabetic or hypertensive middle-aged adult. When investigating older patients arriving at a satisfactory explanation for anemia, particularly mild anemia (hemoglobin 10.5–12 g/dL) is often not successful.

Approximately one-third of anemic older persons lack a clear mechanism accounting for the anemia,[1,5,19,21,26-30] and such individuals are now considered to have UAE. In light of the robust, albeit associative data on the negative implications of even minor anemia (as discussed previously), further examination and eventual interventional trials have become a topic of focused interest in clinical geriatric hematology.

Table 1 Common pathways to anemia in the elderly	
Abbreviation	**Pathway**
Iron Deficiency	IDA
Anemia of chronic disease (anemia of chronic inflammation)	ACD/ACI
Chronic kidney disease	CKD
Vitamin B12/folate deficiency	
Endocrine senescence	Thyroid, androgen
Malnutrition	
Myelodysplasia	MDS
Unexplained anemia of the elderly	UAE

		%	%
Table 2 **Anemia in geriatric populations**			
Study	Population	Anemic	UAE
Guralnik et al,[1] 2004	Community (NHANES III)	11	33
Ble et al,[57] 2005	Community (InCHIANTI)	10	37
Artz and Thirman[44] 2011	Hematology referral, University of Chicago	N/A	44
Price et al,[31] 2011	Hematology referral, Stanford University	N/A	35
Artz et al,[21] 2004	Nursing home, NGRC	49	44

Abbreviations: InCHIANTI, Invecchiare in Chianti, aging in the Chianti area; NGRC, National Geriatrics Research Consortium; NHANES, National Health and Nutrition Examination Survey.

At 2 academic centers within the United States, multidisciplinary clinics are actively addressing key questions regarding UAE (**Table 4**). Investigators at Stanford University developed an aggressive algorithm of laboratory studies to more tightly established the incidence of "unexplained" anemia in the community.[31] Enrolled subjects had been referred for anemia evaluation at either the University or the affiliated Department of Veterans Affairs Hospital hematology clinics. Laboratory testing included a complete blood count with red cell indices, iron indices (serum iron, transferrin saturation, and ferritin), vitamin B12 and folic acid, thyroid-stimulating hormone, erythropoietin level, and serum protein electrophoresis. Additional evaluations were added as clinically indicated and these included bone marrow aspirate and biopsy, interleukin (IL)-6, and hepcidin assays. A similar systematic evaluation of geriatric anemia was undertaken at the University of Chicago. The results summarized in **Table 4** indicate that despite significant demographic differences in subjects evaluated at the 2 different sites, thorough investigation was remarkably similar with regard to identifying a significant subpopulation of anemic patients who did not meet established criteria for a more precise diagnosis than "unexplained anemia."

The Stanford study included a review of the peripheral smear of all patients by each of the investigators. In so doing, they discovered 31 patients (16%) with macrocytic red cells, other cytopenias, and/or dysplastic features considered worrisome for evolving myelodysplasia. In the Chicago study, in which close to 70% of the study participants were African American, the investigators found approximately 5% to meet criteria for thalassemia.

Additional reports from other institutions regarding anemia pathogenesis in the elderly have described iron deficiency in 20%, anemia of chronic disease or inflammation in 15% to 35%, chronic kidney disease in fewer than 10%, and folate/vitamin B12 deficiencies in 10% with a residual subset of approximately one-third UAE.[1,6,21,26,32]

In light of the multitude of adverse outcomes associated with anemia in older patients (mentioned previously) it remains important to pursue serious and/or treatable underlying medical conditions, including iron, folate, or B12 deficiency; blood loss; kidney disease; infection; and hematologic or nonhematologic malignancy (see **Table 3**).

Red blood cell indices may be particularly useful in guiding the anemia workup. Smaller red cells (mean corpuscular volume [MCV] <80 fL) points to iron deficiency, inflammation, chronic disease, or thalassemia, all of which can be confirmed by readily available chemistries or genetic testing if thalassemia is suspected. However, clinicians need to be aware that MCV increases with advancing age[33] and elderly patients may be severely iron deficient despite normal MCV. In elderly patients with large red

Table 3
Laboratory findings in the common anemias of the elderly

Anemia Type	MCV	Iron/TIBC	Ferritin	ESR/CRP	Epo	CrCl	Test	Albumin	Misc
IDA	Small	Low/High	Low	nl	High	nl	nl	nl	
AI/ACD	Small	Low/Low	Low to High	High	Bl	nl	nl	Low to nl	
CKD	nl	nl	nl	nl	Low	<30 mL/min	nl	Low to nl	
Hypothyroid	Large	nl	nl	nl	High	nl	nl	nl	TSH high
B12/folate	Large	nl	nl	nl	High	nl	nl	nl	Vitamin levels low, MMA high
MDS	Large	nl	nl	nl	High	nl	nl	nl	Marrow can be diagnostic
Malnutrition	nl	nl	nl	nl	Bl	nl	Low to nl	Low	
UAE	nl	nl	nl	nl	Bl	nl	Low to nl	nl	

Abbreviations: ACD, anemia of chronic disease; AI, anemia of inflammation; Bl, blunted response (see text); CKD, chronic kidney disease; CrCl, creatinine clearance; CRP, C-reactive protein; Epo, erythropoietin; ESR, erythrocyte sedimentation rate; IDA, iron deficiency anemia; MDS, myelodysplastic syndrome; MMA, methylmalonic acid; nl, normal; TIBC, total iron binding capacity; TSH, thyroid-stimulating hormone; UAE, unexplained anemia of the elderly.

Table 4
Evaluation of geriatric anemia at 2 academic hematology units

	Stanford[31] n = 190	Chicago[44] n = 174
Study similarities	Age (~77 y), prevalent DM, hypertension	
Differences	Mostly male, white, veterans	Mostly female, African American
Anemia Type	**% Stanford**	**% Chicago**
UAE	35	44
IDA	12	25
AI (ACD)	6	10
Heme malignancy	6	7
CKD	4	3
MDS	16	
Thalassemia		5
Other/Incomplete	12	

Abbreviations: ACD, anemia of chronic disease; AI, anemia of inflammation; CKD, chronic kidney disease; DM, diabetes mellitus; IDA, iron deficiency anemia; MDS, myelodysplasia; UAE, unexplained anemia of the elderly.

cells, common causes such as myelodysplasia, B12 deficiency, liver disease, chemotherapy, or alcoholism are to be considered. Peripheral blood smear should be examined for dysplastic features that could indicate underlying myelodysplasia (MDS). Bone marrow sampling using immunohistochemical and molecular/genetic studies might provide diagnostic and therapeutic value for the spectrum of hematologic disorders classified as MDS.[34,35] These studies have become particularly more relevant, as novel and well-tolerated pharmacologic approaches are currently available for older patients with MDS.[36]

Because the hemoglobin threshold below which physical function and overall survival is impaired may be lower for African American compared with white individuals,[24,37] controversy exists about whether the causes of anemia differ sufficiently to justify using a lower hemoglobin threshold to prompt an evaluation in older African American individuals.[24,38]

DEFINING UNEXPLAINED ANEMIA

For the 33% to 50% of geriatric patients with anemia who do not meet standard criteria for anemia subclassification, the diagnosis of UA is becoming increasingly recognized.[39–43] Most commonly, this is a mild, hypoproliferative anemia with hemoglobin levels in the 10 to 12 g/dL range with normocytic indices. Ironically, more severe anemias are rarely difficult to classify. UAE is likely multifactorial, with variable contributions from renal, endocrine deficiency (blunted erythropoietin response), chronic inflammation, androgen deficiency, and possibly nascent myelodysplasia.

Renal Endocrine Deficiency

Despite anemic hemoglobin levels and seemingly normal exocrine function, several series of patients with UAE have demonstrated serum erythropoietin levels significantly lower than expected for degree of anemia.[21,31,44] Of note, although serum erythropoietin levels were shown to rise gradually over time in healthy volunteers enrolled and studied for more than 40 years in the Baltimore Longitudinal Study of Aging (BLSA), those who developed hypertension and/or diabetes while continuing as volunteer BLSA participants were shown to have erythropoietin levels that did not rise but remained stable or even fell. It was these same individuals with stable or dropping erythropoietin levels who developed anemia during their course on the longitudinal study.[45]

Smoldering Inflammation

Despite the absence of clinically apparent acute or chronic inflammatory disease, subjects with UA exhibit markers for low-level smoldering inflammation.[46,47] Furthermore, the degree to which this is present seems to presage several features of frailty, including functional decline and development of age-related disease. Inflammatory markers, such as IL-6 and hepcidin, have been shown to be elevated in most, but not all patients with UAE.[31,44,48]

Androgen Deficiency

Before more modern immunosuppressive therapies and stem cell transplantation, androgens were commonly used to treat aplastic anemia and other hypoplastic marrow conditions.[49] Such treatment was given with the expectation that hemoglobin would rise by 0.8 to 1.0 g/dL. Furthermore, hypogonadal men or those who had been treated with hormonal ablation are typically anemic, with hemoglobin levels frequently 1 g/dL below the lower limit of normal. Because testosterone levels decline with age,[2] Ferrucci and colleagues[50] studied the interaction of testosterone and anemia in a population-based sample of community-dwelling elderly (InCHIANTI study). They found in both older men and women a direct and significant correlation between low testosterone and anemia, either at initial evaluation or at the time of follow-up 3 years later.[50]

Malnutrition

Weight loss and nutritional inadequacy are commonly observed in frail nursing home patients,[51] as is the occurrence of anemia.[52] In a recent research report from Switzerland examining frequency and pathogenesis of anemia in 392 institutionalized elderly, the prevalence of anemia was 39%.[42] After thorough anemia investigation and using multivariate analysis, those who met criteria for anemia were more likely to have low serum albumin and prealbumin levels. Approximately one-third of the anemic patients were classified as UAE and 91% of these had low serum albumin and prealbumin. Thus, markers of malnutrition were strongly associated with anemia in the frail elderly. The investigators concluded that screening for undernutrition should be included in anemia assessment, particularly in frail nursing home patients.

Comorbidity Burden

Michalak and colleagues[53] from Poland highlight another perspective. Comorbidity, a known feature of advancing age,[54,55] was examined in the context of anemia occurrence in a retrospective analysis of 981 patients aged $\geq$60 years seen in a primary care practice over a 2-year span. Of the 981 analyzed patients, 17.2% were anemic and, of these, 28.4% were classified as "unexplained." The study highlighted the importance of repeated hospitalizations and the occurrence of anemia. They found that hospital-acquired anemia was more likely to be apparent in those undergoing invasive medical procedures, excessive testing, and/or who were on anticoagulants. For the study population as a whole, by univariate analysis, patients with 2 to 5 comorbidities had a 2-fold to 14-fold risk of anemia. By multivariate logistic regression, factors increasing the risk of anemia were age $\geq$80 years, the number of comorbidities (2 to 4), and recent hospitalization(s). Accordingly, comorbidity burden and hospitalizations are factors to be considered in both overall anemia and UA in the elderly. For

UAE, one might expect that comorbidities and hospitalizations influence erythropoiesis by associated acquired iron deficiency, acute/chronic inflammation, and malnutrition. Nonetheless, by multivariate analysis with these factors included, comorbidity and hospitalization stood alone as risk factors for anemia.

APPROACH TO ELDERLY PATIENTS WITH ANEMIA

Elderly patients who present with severe anemia (hemoglobin <7 g/dL) most frequently have evidence for acute or chronic bleeding, hemolysis, or bone marrow compromised by hematologic or nonhematologic neoplasia. Workup is prompt, often involving endoscopies or hematologist consultation. However, many elderly patients will more commonly present with moderate or even minor anemia, and workup will reveal characteristics of UA. It is our practice to conduct a standard laboratory evaluation for anemia, including complete blood count with red cell indices and reticulocyte count; and in addition, an assessment of iron, percent transferrin saturation and total iron binding capacity, B12, albumin, total serum protein, serum creatinine, and erythrocyte sedimentation rate. From these studies, approximately 70% of ambulatory anemic patients will be readily classified. The great majority of the remaining 30% will fit current criteria of UA. Some patients with UA will have dysplastic features on their peripheral blood smear, macrocytic red blood cells or other cytopenias, and such patients should be referred to a hematologist for additional studies to confirm suspicion of myelodysplasia or other primary bone marrow disorder.

APPROACH TO MANAGEMENT OF UNEXPLAINED ANEMIA IN THE ELDERLY

There have been no published reports that describe the natural history of UA or whether treatment can ameliorate any of the adverse associations described previously. Nonetheless, the blunted erythropoietin level observed in most patients presents a tempting target for intervention. A well-constructed clinical trial examining the effects of recombinant erythropoietin (eg, Procrit, Aranesp) on hemoglobin level, relevant physical and psychological functions, and safety remains to be conducted. Features of this study should include careful selection of volunteers who meet criteria for UAE and study outcomes other than hemoglobin level alone that include relevant physical function (eg, 6-minute walk), cognition, and quality of life. Further, an optimal study would be of sufficient duration to allow a reasonable chance that sustained improvement in hemoglobin level would favorably influence those outcomes.

Another target for treatment of UA in the elderly includes testosterone replacement. In this regard, a recent multi-institutional randomized trial examining whether testosterone treatment of older men with previously determined low testosterone levels was recently published.[56] Testosterone gel with doses adjusted to maintain testosterone levels in normal range was administered for 12 months. The investigators looked specifically for treatment effect for those subjects with UA. Of 788 enrolled subjects, 126 were anemic, and 62 of these were classified as UA. More than 50% of anemic subjects (total group and specifically UA) had a >1 g/dL rise in hemoglobin by the 12th month of treatment. Despite this encouraging finding, the investigators appropriately pointed out that the overall health benefits of improved hemoglobin level remain to be established.

Other potential targets for UA treatment under consideration include anti-inflammatory strategies (such as hepcidin inhibitors) or nutritional supplements, particularly for frail elderly with established malnutrition.

Although UA is being increasingly recognized and its importance more generally understood, because of its heterogenous pathophysiology, only by well-constructed clinical trials will effective treatment interventions be established.

SUMMARY

The prevalence of anemia increases with advancing age, and despite thorough investigation, approximately one-third will be classified as "unexplained." UA is typically hypoproliferative, normocytic, and with a low reticulocyte count. Serum erythropoietin levels are lower than would be expected for degree of anemia. Chronic inflammation, low testosterone levels, malnutrition, and possibly nascent myelodysplasia are variably contributing factors. No clearly established beneficial treatment strategy has been established, but the association of UA with a wide range of adverse outcomes, including impaired quality of life, physical function, and mortality, is sufficiently compelling to justify expanding clinical research focused on both basic and clinical aspects.

REFERENCES

1. Guralnik JM, Eisenstaedt RS, Ferrucci L, et al. Prevalence of anemia in persons 65 years and older in the United States: evidence for a high rate of unexplained anemia. Blood 2004;104(8):2263–8.
2. Harman SM, Metter EJ, Tobin JD, et al, Baltimore Longitudinal Study of Aging. Longitudinal effects of aging on serum total and free testosterone levels in healthy men. Baltimore Longitudinal Study of Aging. J Clin Endocrinol Metab 2001;86(2):724–31.
3. Gaskell H, Derry S, Andrew Moore R, et al. Prevalence of anaemia in older persons: systematic review. BMC Geriatr 2008;8:1.
4. Ania BJ, Suman VJ, Fairbanks VF, et al. Prevalence of anemia in medical practice: community versus referral patients. Mayo Clin Proc 1994;69(8):730–5.
5. Ania BJ, Suman VJ, Fairbanks VF, et al. Incidence of anemia in older people: an epidemiologic study in a well defined population. J Am Geriatr Soc 1997;45(7):825–31.
6. Ferrucci L, Guralnik JM, Bandinelli S, et al. Unexplained anaemia in older persons is characterised by low erythropoietin and low levels of pro-inflammatory markers. Br J Haematol 2007;136(6):849–55.
7. Chaves PH, Ashar B, Guralnik JM, et al. Looking at the relationship between hemoglobin concentration and prevalent mobility difficulty in older women. Should the criteria currently used to define anemia in older people be reevaluated? J Am Geriatr Soc 2002;50(7):1257–64.
8. Penninx BW, Guralnik JM, Onder G, et al. Anemia and decline in physical performance among older persons. Am J Med 2003;115(2):104–10.
9. Penninx BW, Kritchevsky SB, Newman AB, et al. Inflammatory markers and incident mobility limitation in the elderly. J Am Geriatr Soc 2004;52(7):1105–13.
10. Culleton BF, Manns BJ, Zhang J, et al. Impact of anemia on hospitalization and mortality in older adults. Blood 2006;107(10):3841–6.
11. Hong CH, Falvey C, Harris TB, et al. Anemia and risk of dementia in older adults: findings from the Health ABC study. Neurology 2013;81(6):528–33.
12. Onder G, Penninx BW, Cesari M, et al. Anemia is associated with depression in older adults: results from the InCHIANTI study. J Gerontol A Biol Sci Med Sci 2005;60(9):1168–72.

13. Thein M, Ershler WB, Artz AS, et al. Diminished quality of life and physical function in community-dwelling elderly with anemia. Medicine (Baltimore) 2009;88(2): 107–14.

14. Penninx BW, Pahor M, Cesari M, et al. Anemia is associated with disability and decreased physical performance and muscle strength in the elderly. J Am Geriatr Soc 2004;52(5):719–24.

15. Beghe C, Wilson A, Ershler WB. Prevalence and outcomes of anemia in geriatrics: a systematic review of the literature. Am J Med 2004;116(Suppl 7A):3S–10S.

16. Chaves PH, Xue QL, Guralnik JM, et al. What constitutes normal hemoglobin concentration in community-dwelling disabled older women? J Am Geriatr Soc 2004; 52(11):1811–6.

17. Zakai NA, Katz R, Hirsch C, et al. A prospective study of anemia status, hemoglobin concentration, and mortality in an elderly cohort: the Cardiovascular Health Study. Arch Intern Med 2005;165(19):2214–20.

18. Alkema L, Gerland P, Raftery A, et al. The United Nations probabilistic population projections: an introduction to demographic forecasting with uncertainty. Foresight (Colch) 2015;2015(37):19–24.

19. Sahadevan S, Choo PW, Jayaratnam FJ. Anaemia in the hospitalised elderly. Singapore Med J 1995;36(4):375–8.

20. Steensma DP, Tefferi A. Anemia in the elderly: how should we define it, when does it matter, and what can be done? Mayo Clin Proc 2007;82(8):958–66.

21. Artz AS, Fergusson D, Drinka PJ, et al. Mechanisms of unexplained anemia in the nursing home. J Am Geriatr Soc 2004;52(3):423–7.

22. Robinson B, Artz AS, Culleton B, et al. Prevalence of anemia in the nursing home: contribution of chronic kidney disease. J Am Geriatr Soc 2007;55(10):1566–70.

23. Beutler E, West C. Hematologic differences between African-Americans and whites: the roles of iron deficiency and alpha-thalassemia on hemoglobin levels and mean corpuscular volume. Blood 2005;106(2):740–5.

24. Patel KV, Harris TB, Faulhaber M, et al. Racial variation in the relationship of anemia with mortality and mobility disability among older adults. Blood 2007;109(11): 4663–70.

25. Patel KV, Longo DL, Ershler WB, et al. Haemoglobin concentration and the risk of death in older adults: differences by race/ethnicity in the NHANES III follow-up. Br J Haematol 2009;145(4):514–23.

26. Joosten E, Pelemans W, Hiele M, et al. Prevalence and causes of anaemia in a geriatric hospitalized population. Gerontology 1992;38(1–2):111–7.

27. Kirkeby OJ, Fossum S, Risoe C. Anaemia in elderly patients. Incidence and causes of low haemoglobin concentration in a city general practice. Scand J Prim Health Care 1991;9(3):167–71.

28. McLennan WJ, Andrews GR, Macleod C, et al. Anaemia in the elderly. Q J Med 1973;42(165):1–13.

29. Nilsson-Ehle H, Jagenburg R, Landahl S, et al. Haematological abnormalities and reference intervals in the elderly. A cross-sectional comparative study of three urban Swedish population samples aged 70, 75 and 81 years. Acta Med Scand 1988;224(6):595–604.

30. Nilsson-Ehle H, Jagenburg R, Landahl S, et al. Haematological abnormalities in a 75-year-old population. Consequences for health-related reference intervals. Eur J Haematol 1988;41(2):136–46.

31. Price EA, Mehra R, Holmes TH, et al. Anemia in older persons: etiology and evaluation. Blood Cells Mol Dis 2011;46(2):159–65.

32. Joosten E, Hiele M, Ghoos Y, et al. Diagnosis of iron-deficiency anemia in a hospitalized geriatric population. Am J Med 1991;90(5):653–4.
33. Hoffmann JJ, Nabbe KC, van den Broek NM. Effect of age and gender on reference intervals of red blood cell distribution width (RDW) and mean red cell volume (MCV). Clin Chem Lab Med 2015;53(12):2015–9.
34. Chung SS, Park CY. Aging, hematopoiesis, and the myelodysplastic syndromes. Blood Adv 2017;1(26):2572–8.
35. Steensma DP. How I use molecular genetic tests to evaluate patients who have or may have myelodysplastic syndromes. Blood 2018;132(16):1657–63.
36. Montoro J, Yerlikaya A, Ali A, et al. Improving treatment for myelodysplastic syndromes patients. Curr Treat Options Oncol 2018;19(12):66.
37. Dong X, de Leon CM, Artz A, et al. A population-based study of hemoglobin, race, and mortality in elderly persons. J Gerontol A Biol Sci Med Sci 2008; 63(8):873–8.
38. Artz A, Dong X. Defining anemia by race using epidemiologic data. Blood 2008; 111(5):2941 [author reply: 2].
39. Halawi R, Moukhadder H, Taher A. Anemia in the elderly: a consequence of aging? Expert Rev Hematol 2017;10(4):327–35.
40. Stauder R, Valent P, Theurl I. Anemia at older age: etiologies, clinical implications, and management. Blood 2018;131(5):505–14.
41. Bach V, Schruckmayer G, Sam I, et al. Prevalence and possible causes of anemia in the elderly: a cross-sectional analysis of a large European university hospital cohort. Clin Interv Aging 2014;9:1187–96.
42. Frangos E, Trombetti A, Graf CE, et al. Malnutrition in very old hospitalized patients: a new etiologic factor of anemia? J Nutr Health Aging 2016;20(7):705–13.
43. Michalak SS, Rupa-Matysek J, Gil L. Comorbidities, repeated hospitalizations, and age >/= 80 years as indicators of anemia development in the older population. Ann Hematol 2018;97(8):1337–47.
44. Artz AS, Thirman MJ. Unexplained anemia predominates despite an intensive evaluation in a racially diverse cohort of older adults from a referral anemia clinic. J Gerontol A Biol Sci Med Sci 2011;66(8):925–32.
45. Ershler WB, Sheng S, McKelvey J, et al. Serum erythropoietin and aging: a longitudinal analysis. J Am Geriatr Soc 2005;53(8):1360–5.
46. Ershler WB. Interleukin-6: a cytokine for gerontologists. J Am Geriatr Soc 1993; 41(2):176–81.
47. Ershler WB, Keller ET. Age-associated increased interleukin-6 gene expression, late-life diseases, and frailty. Annu Rev Med 2000;51:245–70.
48. Ferrucci L, Guralnik JM, Woodman RC, et al. Proinflammatory state and circulating erythropoietin in persons with and without anemia. Am J Med 2005; 118(11):1288.
49. Shahidi NT, Diamond LK. Testosterone-induced remission in aplastic anemia of both acquired and congenital types. Further observations in 24 cases. N Engl J Med 1961;264:953–67.
50. Ferrucci L, Maggio M, Bandinelli S, et al. Low testosterone levels and the risk of anemia in older men and women. Arch Intern Med 2006;166(13):1380–8.
51. Cereda E, Pedrolli C, Klersy C, et al. Nutritional status in older persons according to healthcare setting: a systematic review and meta-analysis of prevalence data using MNA((R)). Clin Nutr 2016;35(6):1282–90.
52. Artz AS, Fergusson D, Drinka PJ, et al. Prevalence of anemia in skilled-nursing home residents. Arch Gerontol Geriatr 2004;39(3):201–6.

53. Michalak SS, Rupa-Matysek J, Gil L. Comorbidities, repeated hospitalizations, and age > 80 years as indicators of anemia development in the older population. Ann Hematol 2018;97(8):1337–47.
54. Barnett K, Mercer SW, Norbury M, et al. Epidemiology of multimorbidity and implications for health care, research, and medical education: a cross-sectional study. Lancet 2012;380(9836):37–43.
55. Yancik R, Ershler W, Satariano W, et al. Report of the National Institute on Aging task force on comorbidity. J Gerontol A Biol Sci Med Sci 2007;62(3):275–80.
56. Roy CN, Snyder PJ, Stephens-Shields AJ, et al. Association of testosterone levels with anemia in older men: a controlled clinical trial. JAMA Intern Med 2017; 177(4):480–90.
57. Ble A, Fink JC, Woodman RC, et al. Renal function, erythropoietin, and anemia of older persons: the InCHIANTI study. Arch Intern Med 2005;165(19):2222–7.

Treatment of Iron Deficiency in the Elderly: A New Paradigm

Michael Auerbach, MD[a,b],*, Jerry Spivak, MD[c]

KEYWORDS

- Anemia • Iron deficiency • Intravenous iron • Erythropoiesis

KEY POINTS

- Anemia in the elderly is common.
- Although multifactorial, iron deficiency remains the most common cause.
- Oral iron is poorly tolerated in the majority and is often ineffective due to comorbidities.
- Intravenous iron is underutilized.
- The danger of intravenous iron is misinterpreted and it is much safer than physicians realize.

INTRODUCTION

Aging is associated with an increasing prevalence of mild anemia (<13.2 g/dL of hemoglobin in men and <12.2 g/dL in women),[1] such that approximately 10% of community-dwelling individuals older than 65 years are anemic.[2,3] This is not a trivial statistic; rather, it is one with important implications for public health and medical economics in this expanding population cohort, currently approximately 15% of the US population and much higher in developing countries. In this aging population, even mild anemia is associated with impaired physical and cognitive function,[4] decreased quality of life, increased hospital admissions, prolonged hospital stays,[5] and increased mortality.[6–8] Importantly, the aging process per se cannot be directly implicated in the development of anemia. The hemoglobin distribution curves for healthy individuals over age 65 are similar to younger age groups for both genders. In a study of healthy, community-dwelling adults aged 84 years and older, red blood cell values were similar to those in a cohort of younger adults except for slightly lower hemoglobin, red cell

Disclosure Statement: Dr M. Auerbach has received research funding for data management from AMAG. J. Spivak has nothing to disclose.
[a] Auerbach Hematology and Oncology, 5233 King Avenue #308, Baltimore, MD 21237, USA;
[b] Georgetown University School of Medicine, Washington, DC, USA; [c] Johns Hopkins University School of Medicine, 720 Rutland Avenue, Baltimore, MD 21205, USA
* Corresponding author. Auerbach Hematology and Oncology, 5233 King Avenue #308, Baltimore, MD 21237.
E-mail address: mauerbachmd@abhemonc.com

count values, and mean corpuscular volume (MCV) elevation in the older men but still within the range of normal,[9] which is probably explained by age-related reduction in testosterone production.

Androgen deprivation in men results in a fall in hemoglobin of approximately 1 g/dL without a change in the serum erythropoietin level but with a slight increase in the red cell MCV,[10] which is compatible with the gradual decline in hemoglobin observed in men after age 70 but never below normal.[11] In this regard, neither the serum erythropoietin level nor its production in response to anemia are impaired in the healthy elderly,[12] and the erythropoietic response of the bone marrow to recombinant erythropoietin therapy is normal. The concept that aging restricts erythropoiesis is also refuted by the robust erythroid response of the bone marrow in elderly patients who acquire the myeloproliferative neoplasm polycythemia vera.

Although acquisition of mutations in genes, such as DNM3TA and TET2, increases with age (age-related clonal hematopoiesis)[13] and can promote clonal hematopoietic stem cell expansion, such clones typically are small and do not influence blood cell counts in most individuals. The production of inflammatory cytokines, including interleukin (IL)-6 and IL-1β, and the inflammatory markers C-reactive protein and fibrinogen increases in the elderly, primarily after age 75,[14] but, surprisingly, hepcidin levels are not elevated,[15] indicating a poor correlation between inflammatory markers and anemia in the elderly.

With respect to causes of anemia in the US elderly community-dwelling population, the Third National Health and Nutritional Examination Survey (NHANES III) identified 3 major categories: nutritional (deficiencies of iron, folic acid, or vitamin B_{12}, alone or in combination); renal insufficiency and/or the anemia of chronic inflammation (ACI); and unexplained anemia (UA).[2] Both the ACI and UA populations were associated with multiple comorbidities, including diabetes, hypertension, congestive heart failure, arthritis, and cancer but most commonly with the UA population. In this regard, the prevalence and causes of anemia in the hospitalized elderly is informative with respect to their community-dwelling counterparts.[5] Overall, the prevalence of anemia was 58% and greater in patients older than 65 than those younger (62% to 44%), whereas the severity of anemia was mild in 57% of the patients. The distribution of causes was in part similar to the NHANES III categories (nutritional, renal, and ACI), including the association with multiple comorbidities, with the exceptions of 2 additional categories, hemorrhage and hematologic malignancies or solid tumors; in contrast to the community-dwelling elderly, a cause for anemia was not found in only 5%. A significant association with age was found only for the anemia of chronic renal failure.

The distribution of anemia categories between the community-dwelling and hospitalized population studies cannot accounted for by population age differences, rather in part to the presence of malignancies and a greater prevalence of chronic renal failure in the hospitalized elderly population. This, however, does not totally account for unidentified anemia in the community-dwelling elderly population. The explanation involves a redefinition of ACI. The anemia associated with aging in the absence of active blood loss is hypoproliferative in nature regardless of cause. Exact diagnosis is difficult because the hallmarks of its most common nutritional cause, iron deficiency, are masked by the accumulated comorbidities of the aging process, which also may prevent its correction.[5] Thus, the classic categories of anemia, microcytic, normocytic, and macrocytic, are not useful in the elderly. Instead, it is more appropriate to evaluate anemia based on the 4 essential factors for erythropoiesis: the functional capacity of the bone marrow; the available nutrients; the intensity for the stimulus for red cell production; and red cell life span. As discussed previously, aging does not per se impair bone marrow function and red cell life span is normal. With a normal fortified diet and gastrointestinal absorptive function, the fundamental rate-limiting process in erythropoiesis is stimulation by erythropoietin, which also not is impacted by age.

Two processes have an impact on the production of erythropoietin: increased and impaired intracellular iron in erythropoietin-producing cells, which, like oxygen, accelerates the destruction of hypoxia inducible factor-1/2α, the regulators of erythropoietin gene expression, and impaired renal endocrine function. The tissue sequestration of iron associated with inflammation, infection, and cancer (ACI) accounts for the first process, whereas subclinical impairment of renal endocrine function out of proportion to renal excretory function due to diabetes, long-standing hypertension, inflammation, or cardiac disease accounts for the second.[2,16–18] Although, erythropoietin production is most severely depressed at a creatinine clearance less than 30 mL/min, it is also progressively depressed as the creatinine clearance falls below normal (60 mL/min).[19] Thus, it is likely that most of the unexplained cases of mild anemia in the aged in NHANES III were a consequence of impaired renal erythropoietin production.[20]

Iron deficiency is the most common nutritional cause of the anemia associated with aging, accounting for approximately 17% of anemia.[2] In the elderly, as in their younger counterparts, the gastrointestinal tract seems the principal site of blood loss, with peptic ulceration and cancer the leading causes; in elderly women, bleeding causes outnumber nonbleeding causes, such as celiac disease and atrophic gastritis or helicobacter-induced gastritis.[21] In the elderly, with respect to occult bleeding, in addition to cancer, colonic angiodysplasia is a cause often difficult to establish diagnostically. In hospitalized patients, iatrogenic iron deficiency due to diagnostic phlebotomies always must be considered. Lack of response to iron therapy may be due to the route chosen for iron administration, concomitant vitamin B_{12} deficiency, continued occult bleeding, or impairment of erythropoietin production due to impaired renal erythropoietin production out of proportion to renal excretory function, and these issues are the subject of this article.

Anemia adds to morbidity and mortality across a wide gamut of medical conditions, and its treatment is often marginalized by practitioners, considering it a subclinical variant of aging. As is the case in younger individuals, iron deficiency plays a major causative role. Unlike a younger population, however, comorbid conditions frequently, if not usually, cause iron-restricted erythropoiesis, impairing the current standard of administering oral iron as frontline therapy.

As in younger adults, the most common cause of anemia is iron deficiency.[22] If uncomplicated and mild, oral iron remains the recommended up-front therapy. High-quality evidence, however, reports greater than 70% of those to whom it is prescribed reporting significant gastrointestinal perturbation, with low adherence to prescribed therapy.[23] The most frequent of these adverse events is worsening constipation, which is much more common in the individuals over the age of 60 in whom bowel motility is decreased. Furthermore, serum ferritin levels as well as serum hepcidin levels increase with age, decreasing both iron absorption and utilization. In normal individuals, approximately 10% of ingested iron, either in food or pills, is absorbed. This limitation of enteral iron's benefit is complicated further by recent high-quality evidence reporting increased hepcidin levels after the ingestion of oral iron supplementation, resulting in decreased absorption of daily or twice-daily ferrous sulfate compared with an every-other-day schedule.[24,25]

This article focuses on the etiology and treatment of iron deficiency in the aged. The authors hope to provide a cogent argument for a shift in the current paradigm of using oral iron as the preferred route of replacement to parenteral iron, which has been shown to be safe, better tolerated, more effective, and more convenient to both patients and providers.

DIAGNOSIS

A low hemoglobin concentration with microcytic indices and a low reticulocyte count are considered classic findings. In iron deficiency anemia, however, the hemoglobin falls prior to the indices, which may remain normal for protracted periods if the equilibrium with dietary intake remains close to normal.[26] Subsequently, waiting for anemia or microcytosis to occur may miss a substantial portion of iron-deficient individuals and delay a diagnosis of a potentially dangerous cause of blood loss.

While awaiting clinical outcome validation of newer tests for making the diagnosis of iron deficiency, such as the transferrin receptor, transferrin receptor/serum ferritin index, and reticulocyte hemoglobin content (CHr), as of this writing the most widely utilized iron parameters are the serum ferritin and the percent saturation of transferrin. A serum ferritin below the lower limit of normal is diagnostic of iron deficiency; however, the use of the ferritin is complicated by its acute-phase reactivity and normal levels by no means rule out the diagnosis. The lower limit of normal for serum ferritin is usually stated as 20 ng/mL to 30 ng/mL, but most investigators agree in the presence of comorbidities, ferritin levels below 100 ng/mL usually are considered consistent with iron lack. The serum iron and the total iron-binding capacity are used to calculate the percent saturation of transferrin (TSAT). Values below 20% and certainly below 18% suggest an inadequate supply of iron for erythropoiesis. A very low value (<15%) is characteristic of iron deficiency.[27] A low TSAT currently remains the most reliable indicator of iron need and in the authors' practice informs treatment.

The CHr promises to be a rapidly available test to define a need for iron replacement. The CHr is a snapshot of recent iron availability for hemoglobin synthesis.[27] In iron deficiency the CHr is low but it is also low in a variety of other conditions associated with impaired iron availability (iron-restricted erythropoiesis). The measurement of the CHr is currently on some autoanalyzers and has been shown to predict the need for iron replacement as well as response to therapy (Carlo Brugnara, MD, Harvard Medical School, personal communication, 2018). Although the authors eagerly look forward to the publication and validation of this data, the TSAT remains the current standard to inform iron need.

SIGNS AND SYMPTOMS OF IRON DEFICIENCY

Fatigue is a ubiquitous symptom but it is nonspecific. Further iron deficiency, independent of anemia, may lead to fatigue. Pagophagia (ice craving) or other forms of pica and/or restless legs syndrome[28] are present in at least 50% of those with iron deficiency, with or without anemia, and respond with dramatic alacrity to therapy. If a trial of oral or parenteral iron alleviates these commonly seen symptoms, it is virtually diagnostic. Commonly seen physical findings include pallor, which is nonspecific, a decreased papillation of the tongue, cracking of the corners of the mouth (cheilosis), and prominent defects of the nail beds (koilonychia). If pica is present, much more common in younger women and children for unexplained reasons, because of its vagueness and chronicity, history taking must be specific.

TREATMENT OF IRON DEFICIENCY IN THE ELDERLY

Transient causes of blood loss leading to iron deficiency are common in the elderly. Although it is implicit to search for the etiology, the work-up and diagnosis of bleeding are beyond the scope of this review. Peptic ulcers, bleeding diverticula, angiodysplasia, and other causes of arteriovenous malformations are common, especially in elderly diabetics, which may lead to occult blood loss making the diagnosis problematic. If the etiology of the iron deficiency can be treated and eliminated and there are no underlying comorbidities, it is appropriate and reasonable to prescribe oral iron. Sydenham first used iron filings in cold wine in 1681[29] to treat the "green sickness," later termed "chlorosis" by Blaud, in 1832,[30] who was the first to use ferrous sulfate (although a variety of newer formulations, including carbonyl iron, ferric citrate, polysaccharide-iron complex, and heme iron, have been touted to be either better tolerated and/or more effective than ferrous sulfate, none has proved superior in prospective studies). By the time of the American Civil War, oral iron was used to treat wounds and today iron deficiency is the most common micronutrient deficiency on the planet, estimated to affect more than 35% of the world's population, or approximately 3 billion people.[31] Ferrous sulfate is inexpensive, widely available, and, if tolerated, effective. Unfortunately, oral iron is rife with side effects, including nausea, gastric cramping, diarrhea, and worsening constipation, a frequent unrelated preexisting condition in the elderly.[32] Therefore, more than 300 years later, oral iron, often ineffective and usually poorly tolerated, is used as the frontline treatment of the most common malady on earth. A new treatment paradigm is proposed.

In a prospective, randomized study of different doses of oral iron in elderly iron-deficient individuals, Rimon and colleagues,[33] randomized 90 patients with iron deficiency to 15 mg, 50 mg, or 150 mg of liquid ferrous gluconate per day and concluded that low-dose iron treatment is effective in elderly patients with iron deficiency anemia with fewer side effects. Nonetheless, in the analysis, 46% reported gastrointestinal side effects, including abdominal discomfort, nausea, vomiting, and diarrhea. Curiously, worsening constipation was not seen in the low-dose arm compared with 10% and 23%, respectively, in the higher-dose arms. These results do not include 7% who dropped out and 44% who reported thickened and darkened stools. Darkened stools are unpleasant for older patients and could be mistaken for melena.

More problematic with the use of oral iron is its inability to overcome the iron-restricted erythropoiesis caused by elevated hepcidin levels in myriad conditions commonly observed in an aging population. Hepcidin, the hepatic synthesized iron regulatory protein, irreversibly binds to intracellular ferroportin, the only known cellular iron export protein in humans.[34] Oral iron, unlike intravenous iron, is unable to provide a quantitatively significant amount of iron and its benefit subsequently is suboptimal. In contradistinction, intravenous iron is able to bypass this block by skipping the need for absorption by the small intestinal epithelium, which is known to be inhibited by hepcidin. After an injection of intravenous iron, circulating macrophages well known to be extremely avid for iron, take up residual circulating iron not bound to transferrin. When iron gets into the macrophage, it up-regulates iron regulatory proteins 1 and 2, which in turn up-regulate the synthesis of ferroportin, overcoming, at least in part, the hepcidin block. Although unproved by in vitro studies, the dramatic decrement in erythropoiesis-stimulating agent doses as well as time to desired hemoglobin targets achieved by intravenous, and not oral, iron in the anemia of chronic kidney disease and the anemia of cancer and cancer chemotherapy provides strong support for this hypothesis.

INTRAVENOUS IRON

The earliest formulations of intravenous iron were iron colloids and associated with severe side effects due to release of large amounts of labile free iron, leading to a virtual proscription of its use. In 1954, a solution of iron dextran was introduced by Baird and Padmore.[35] With its much more complex carbohydrate core, iron dextran allowed a large dose of iron to be administered without the dangerous hemodynamic adverse events seen with the colloidal formulations. Nearly ubiquitous clinical benefit was observed but hypersensitivity reactions leading to anaphylaxis, although uncommon, hampered its adoption. The first American study on the use of iron dextran was published in 1964[36]; 37 patients with iron deficiency anemia and oral iron intolerance were treated with a total dose infusion of a high-molecular-weight iron dextran (Imferon, Fisons, Holmes Chapel, England). All responded but 2 had self-limited signs of minor infusion reactions and no serious adverse events were observed. Nonetheless it was not until 1980 when the next American study of the use of intravenous iron was published[37]; 471 iron-deficient adults were treated with a total dose infusion of the same high-molecular-weight iron dextran. Seven had signs of hypersensitivity, considered anaphylactoid. There were no deaths or residua and all responded. The investigators concluded that intravenous iron be reserved for those extreme circumstances when iron replacement was urgent and oral iron could not be used. Intravenous iron remained a minor product with limited use.

Then, in 1989, recombinant human erythropoietin was released for use in dialysis-associated anemia providing an obligate need for intravenous iron. In 1991, Imferon was removed from markets worldwide and low-molecular-weight iron dextran was released for use for the dialysis population. Until 1996, iron dextran was associated with only rare adverse events, when another high-molecular-weight iron dextran (Dexferrum, American Regent/Luitpold, Shirley, New York) was released. Safety concerns continued with this new formulation and reports of anaphylaxis dramatically increased.[38] In 1999 and 2000, 2 iron salts, ferric gluconate and iron sucrose, were approved for use in patients with chronic kidney disease, ostensibly associated with fewer adverse events than iron dextran. In 2006, however, Chertow and colleagues[39] retrospectively analyzing more than 30 million doses of intravenous iron, concluded that virtually all serious adverse events were due to the high-molecular-weight formulation and recommended its avoidance and concluded that when high-molecular-weight iron dextran is avoided the other formulations are safe, with an estimated incidence of serious adverse events of less than 1:250,000 administrations. In 2009, high-molecular-weight iron dextran was removed from markets. This conclusion was supported by multiple prospective, retrospective, and intra-institutional observational studies. Sadly, the perception of danger remains today.

Supporting the safety of intravenous iron, are a high quality meta-analysis[40] and an intrainstitutional meta-analysis at the Harvard hospitals.[41] Reporting on the results of studies comprising 10,391 patients, Avni and colleagues[40] compared adverse events in 4044 who received oral iron, 1329 with no iron, 3335 with placebo, and 155 who received intramuscular iron (intramuscular iron is painful, stains the buttock, requires multiple injections without a safety or efficacy advantage, and has been associated with gluteal sarcomas; it should be avoided). Overall, although minor infusion reactions were reported with intravenous iron, there was no increase in serious adverse events compared with any parameter, including placebo. Among the formulations, no difference in safety or efficacy was observed. Corroborating these findings, Okam and colleagues[41] reviewed all the doses of intravenous iron administered at the Harvard hospitals. Consistent with the preponderance of published evidence, when high-molecular-weight iron dextran was excluded, there were no differences in safety among the remaining formulations.

Although there is a dearth of evidence on the specific use of intravenous iron in the elderly, Price and colleagues[42] prospectively evaluated older adults with UA and serum ferritin levels between 20 ng/mL and 200 ng/mL. Intravenous iron sucrose was administered as five injections one week apart is better either immediately after enrollment or after a 12-week wait list period. The primary outcome was change in the 6-minute walk test. Although accrual was difficult and the study was terminated after only 19 subjects enrolled, a significant increment in the 6-minute walk test was observed for those treated immediately and decreased in those delayed, suggesting a subgroup of elderly adults with UA may respond to intravenous iron. No significant toxicity was reported. These results corroborate a previously published prospective, randomized study comparing intravenous iron to oral iron or placebo in patients with chemotherapy-induced anemia receiving erythropoietin,[43] in which the mean age was 66. Whereas intravenous iron markedly decreased time to target hemoglobin levels and resulted in a decrement in erythropoietin dosing, unlike oral iron, which was associated with a 70% incidence of gastrointestinal adverse events, no significant gastrointestinal toxicity with intravenous iron was reported nor were any serious adverse events observed.

A NEW PARADIGM FOR THE TREATMENT OF IRON DEFICIENCY IN THE ELDERLY

Oral iron remains the frontline standard for uncomplicated iron deficiency in which the etiology has been corrected and the treatment is tolerated. Due to the recent evidence that oral iron raises hepcidin with subsequent decrements in absorption, the authors recommend alternate-day dosing. There are several exceptions to this recommendation. For those who have undergone bariatric surgery mitigating the exposure of the oral formulation to gastric acid, which is necessary to conjugate the iron to vitamin C, amino acids, and sugars to protect it from the massive pancreatic alkaline secretions, which otherwise convert it to ferric hydroxide (rust), which cannot be absorbed, should be proscribed (**Fig. 1**). For those with inflammatory bowel disease, active or inactive, the authors recommend the proscription of oral iron due to its direct toxic effect on the intestinal epithelium[44] and alteration of the intestinal bacterial growth having a negative impact on the microbiome.[45]

The choice of intravenous iron formulation is informed by the etiology of the iron deficiency. **Table 1** provides a list of the available formulations in the United States and Europe. With the exception of patients on dialysis or those with chemotherapy-induced anemia in whom frequent visits are necessary as part of the treatment of the underlying disorder, the authors recommend the avoidance of iron sucrose and ferric gluconate due to the multiple visits necessary to complete a treatment course, which add to cost and inconvenience to both patient and provider, without any advantage in either safety or efficacy. Using either of the iron salts quadruples or quintuples the chances for minor infusion reactions and extravasation along with the need to make multiple trips to the infusion center. For all other conditions a single, total dose infusion of either low-molecular-weight iron dextran over 1 hour, or ferumoxytol, ferric carboxymaltose, or iron isomaltoside over 15 minutes, is preferred. By doing so, 1 office visit from 15 minutes to 60 minutes accomplishes what months to more than a

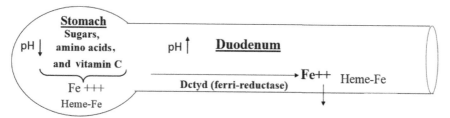

Fig. 1. Iron absorption. (*Courtesy of* Jerry Spivak, MD, Johns Hopkins University School of Medicine, Baltimore, MD.)

Table 1 Intravenous iron preparations				Europe only
Trade name	Infed	Feraheme	Injectafer	Monofer
Manufacturer	Allergan (Chicago, IL)	AMAG Pharmaceuticals (Newton, MA)	Luitpold Pharmaceuticals (Shirley, NY)	Pharmacosmos (Holbaek, Denmark)
Carbohydrate	Low-molecular-weight iron dextran	Ferumoxytol	Carboxymaltose	Isomaltoside
Total dose infusion	Yes	No	Yes	Yes
Test dose required	Yes	No	No	No
Recommended dose	1000 mg	510 mg ×2	750 mg ×2	1000 mg
Infusion time	1 hour	15 min	15 min	15 min
Black box warning	Yes	Yes	No	NA

year of oral iron would require without any of the gastrointestinal perturbation. Minor infusion reactions consisting of pressure in the chest or back or flushing in the face occur in approximately 1% and are self-limited and do not require intervention. The authors normally empirically premedicate with methylprednisolone before rechallenge based on prospective, double-blind evidence reporting its benefit in alleviating the delayed arthralgias and myalgias that occur the next day in the minor or subjects.[46] It is important not to intervene with vasopressors or antihistamines, which can convert these minor, self-limited reactions into serious adverse events ostensibly attributable to the intravenous iron.

As with any intravenous medication, interventions for severe acute hypersensitivity should be available on site. Insurance verification should be obtained prior to administration of any of the formulations because approvals vary.

SUMMARY

Anemia in the elderly is multifactorial. Despite changes in erythropoiesis due to maturation defects, such as myelodysplastic syndrome, chronic kidney disease, and other co-morbid conditions, iron deficiency remains the most common etiology. Oral iron remains the frontline standard when tolerated in the absence of comorbidities mitigating its benefit. In all other clinical circumstances, the intravenous route is preferred. For physicians managing anemia in older patients, familiarity with the available intravenous formulations, their safety, and methods of administration is necessary to provide optimal care.

REFERENCES

1. Beutler E, Waalen J. The definition of anemia: what is the lower limit of normal of the blood hemoglobin concentration? Blood 2006;107:1747–50.
2. Guralnik N, Eisenstaedt R, Ferrucci L, et al. Prevalence of anemia in persons 65 years and older in the United States: evidence for a high rate of unexplained anemia. Blood 2004;104:2263–8.
3. Ageno W, Dentali F, Squizzato A. How I treat splanchinic vein thrombosis. Blood 2014;124:3685–91.

4. Atkinson H, Cesari M, Kritchevsky S, et al. Predictors of combined congitive and physical decline. J Am Geriatr Soc 2005;53:1197–202.

5. Zaninetti C, Klersy C, Scavariello C, et al. Prevalence of anemia in hospitalized internal medicine patients: correlations with comorbidities and length of hospital stay. Eur J Intern Med 2018;51:11–7.

6. Zakai N, French B, Arnold A, et al. Hemoglobin decline, function and mortality in the elderly: the cardiovascular health study. Am J Hematol 2013;88:5–9.

7. Izaks G, Westendorp R, Knook D. The definition of anemia in older persons. JAMA 1999;281:1714–7.

8. Ania B, Suman V, Fairbanks V, et al. Incidence of anemia in older people: an epidemiologic study in a well-defined population. J Am Geriatr Soc 1997;45:825–31.

9. Zauber N, Zauber A. Hematologic data of healthy very old people. JAMA 1987;257:2181–4.

10. Weber J, Walsh P, Peters C, et al. Effect of reversible androgen deprivation on hemoglobin and serum immunoreactive erythropoietin in men. Am J Hematol 1991;36:190–4.

11. Nilsson-Ehle H, Jagenburg R, Landahl S, et al. Blood haemoglobin declines in the elderly: implications for reference intervals age 70 to 88. Eur J Haematol 2000;65:297–305.

12. Powers J, Krantz S, Collins J, et al. Erythropoietin response to anemia as a function of age. J Am Geriatr Soc 1991;39:30–2.

13. Buscarlet M, Provost S, Zada Y, et al. DNMT3A and TET2 dominate clonal hematopoiesis and demonstrate benign phenotypes and different genetic predispositions. Blood 2017;130:753–62.

14. Ferrucci L, Corsi A, Lauretani F, et al. The origins of age-related proinflammatory state. Blood 2005;105:2294–9.

15. Ferrucci L, Semba R, Guralnik J, et al. Proinflammatory state, hepcidin, and anemia in older persons. Blood 2010;115:3810–6.

16. Rarick M, Espina B, Colley D, et al. Treatment of unique anemia in patients with IDDM with epoetin alfa. Diabetes Care 1998;21:423–6.

17. Ferrucci L, Guralnik J, Woodman R, et al. Proinflammatory state and circulating erythropoietin in persons with and without anemia. Am J Med 2005;118:1288.

18. Cash J, Sears D. The anemia of chronic disease: spectrum of associated diseases n series of unselected hospitalized patients. Am J Med 1989;87:638–44.

19. Anpalahan M, Savvas S, Lo K, et al. Chronic idiopathic normocytic anaemia in older people: the risk factors and the role of age-associated renal impairment. Aging Clin Exp Res 2017;29:147–55.

20. Gowanlock Z, Sriram S, Martin A, et al. Erythropoietin levels in elderly patients with anemia of unknown etiology. PLoS One 2016;11:e0157279.

21. Annibale B, Capurso G, Chistolini A, et al. Gastrointestinal causes of refractory iron deficiency anemia in patients without gastrointestinal symptoms. Am J Med 2001;111:439–45.

22. Nahon S, Lahmek P, Aras N, et al. Management and predictors of early mortality in elderly patients with iron deficiency anemia: a prospective study of 111 patients. Gastroenterol Clin Biol 2007;31:169.

23. Tolkien Z, Stecher L, Mander A, et al. Ferrous sulfate supplementation causes significant gastrointestinal side-effects in adults: a systematic review and meta-analysis. PLoS One 2015;10(2):e0117383.

24. Moretti D, Goede J, Zeder C, et al. Oral iron supplements increase hepcidin and decease iron absorption from daily or twice-daily doses in iron-depleted young women. Blood 2015;126:1981–9.
25. Stoffel N, Cercamondi C, Brittenham G, et al. Iron absorption from oral iron supplements given on consecutive versus alternate days and as single morning doses versus twice-daily split dosing in iron-depleted women: two open-label, randomized controlled trials. Lancet Haematol 2017;4:e524–33.
26. Schultz B, Freedman M. Iron deficiency in the elderly. Baillieres Clin Haematol 1987;1:291–313.
27. Auerbach M, Adamson J. How we diagnose and treat iron deficiency anemia. Am J Hematol 2015;91:31–8.
28. Mehmood T, Auerbach M, Earley C, et al. Response to intravenous iron in patients with restless legs syndrome (Willis-Ekbom disease). Sleep Med 2014;15:1473–6.
29. Stockman R. The treatment of chlorosis with iron and some other drugs. Br Med J 1893;1:881–5.
30. Blaud P. Sur les maladies chloropiques et sur un mode de traitement specifique dons ces affecions. Rev Med Fr Etrang 1832;45:357–67.
31. Kassebaum N, Rashmi J, Naghavi M, et al. A systematic analysis of global anemia burden from 1990 to 2010. Blood 2014;123:615–24.
32. Price E, Schrier S. Anemia in the older adult. In: Tirnauer J, Mentzer W, editors. UpToDate. Waltham (MA): UpToDate; 2017.
33. Rimon E, Kagansky N, Kagansky M, et al. Ae we giving too much iron? Low-dose iron therapy is effective in octogenarians. Am J Med 2005;118:1142–7.
34. Camaschella C. The Ham Wasserman Lecture. Iron and hepcidin: a story of recycling and balance. Hematology Am Soc Hematol Educ Program 2013;2013: 1–8.
35. Baird I, Podmore D. Intra-muscular iron therapy in iron deficiency anemia. Lancet 1954;2:942–6.
36. Marchasin S, Wallterstein R. The treatment of iron-deficiency anemia with intravenous iron dextran. Blood 1964;23:354–8.
37. Hamstra R, Block M, Shocket A. Intravenous iron dextran in clinical medicine. JAMA 1980;243:1726–31.
38. Auerbach M, Ballard H. Clinical use of intravenous iron: administration, efficacy, and safety. Hematology Am Soc Hematol Educ Program 2010;2010:338–47.
39. Chertow G, Mason P, Vaage-Nilsen O, et al. Update on adverse drug events associated with parenteral iron. Nephrol Dial Transplant 2006;21:378–82.
40. Avni T, Bieber A, Grossman A, et al. The safety of intravenous iron peparations: systematic review and meta-analysis. Mayo Clin Proc 2015;90:12–23.
41. Okam M, Mandell E, Hevelone N, et al. Comparative rates of adverse events with different formulations of intravenous iron. Am J Hematol 2012;87:e123–4.
42. Price E, Artz A, Barnhart H, et al. A prospective randomized wait list control trial of intravenous iron sucrose in older adults with unexplained anemia and serum ferritin 20-200 ng/mL. Blood Cells Mol Dis 2014;53:221–30.
43. Auerbach M, Ballard H, Trout J, et al. Intravenous iron optimizes the response to recombinant human erythropoietin in cancer patients with chemotherapy-related anemia: results of a multicenter, open-label, randomized trial. J Clin Oncol 2004; 22:1301–7.
44. Gasche C, Lomer M, Cavill I, et al. Iron, anaemia, and inflammatory bowel diseases. Gut 2004;53:1190–7.

45. Lee T, Cavel T, Smirnov K, et al. Oral versus intravenous iron replacement therapy distinctly alters the gut microbiota and metabolome in patients with IBD. Gut 2016;66:863–71.
46. Auerbach M, Chaudhry M, Goldman H, et al. The value of methylprednisolone in prevention of the arthralgia-myalgia syndrome associated with the total dose infusion of iron dextran: a double blind randomized trial. J Lab Clin Med 1998;131: 257–60.

Late Life Vitamin B12 Deficiency

Chad Zik, MD

KEYWORDS

- Vitamin B12 • Elderly patients • Anemia

KEY POINTS

- Vitamin B12 deficiency can present with a wide array of symptoms, and, if unrecognized, lead to significant morbidity especially with regard to the hematologic and neurologic complications.
- Vitamin B12 is far more prevalent in the elderly population than in the general population.
- In particular, the elderly are at higher risk of vitamin B12 deficiency due to higher incidence of polypharmacy, pernicious anemia and food cobalamin malabsorption.

INTRODUCTION

Vitamin B12 deficiency may present with a wide array of symptoms and, if unrecognized, lead to significant morbidity particularly in terms of the hematologic and neurologic complications. This is of particular concern in the elderly because of its high prevalence with advancing age and the enhanced difficulty of recognizing subtle changes in symptoms and distinguishing those from normal aging.

In general, vitamin B12 is available only through the consumption of animal products, including meat, eggs, and dairy. Once vitamin B12 is consumed, it is bound to R protein present in saliva and gastric secretions. Subsequently, intrinsic factor, which is produced by the parietal cells of the stomach, binds to vitamin B12, until it is reabsorbed by the distal ileum.[1]

Once bioavailable, vitamin B12 is used for purine and pyrimidine synthesis and subsequent formation of DNA; deficiency of vitamin B12 can result in arrest in the S phase of cellular division inhibiting further replication.[2] Metabolically, vitamin B12 is required to synthesize methionine from homocysteine in the methionine cycle and in the conversion of methylmalonyl coenzyme A to succinyl coenzyme A.[3] In these pathways, B12 deficiency leads to increases of methylmalonic acid (MMA) and homocysteine.

Disclosure: The author has nothing to disclose.
Virginia Commonwealth University School of Medicine Inova Campus, 8501 Arlington Boulevard, Suite 340, Fairfax, VA 22031, USA
E-mail address: chad.zik@inova.org

The daily requirement of B12 consumption recommended by the US Food and Drug Administration and the Institute of Medicine is 2.4 µg/d[4] for adults, and 2.0 µg/d after 50 years of age.[4] Typical consumption by the average American exceeds this value.[4] Once consumed it is stored hepatically (with stores as high as 1.5 mg); these stores can supply sufficient vitamin B12 for metabolism for 5 to 10 years before deficiency manifests.[5,6]

The elderly have a higher prevalence of B12 deficiency than the general population.[4] Possible reasons for this include decreased gastrin and subsequent decreased gastric acidity, and the increased use of medications that decrease B12 absorption. However, thus far, the available evidence to support these mechanisms has been conflicting.[4]

COBALAMIN (VITAMIN B12) DEFICIENCY

Vitamin B12 (cobalamin) deficiency in the elderly is likely to be more frequent than commonly appreciated. Data from the Framingham study showed that 12% of community-dwelling elderly were cobalamin deficient.[7] Other studies report that as many as 30% to 40% of sick or institutionalized elderly are cobalamin deficient.[8] In one large series from France, nearly 5% of hospitalized patients between the ages of 65 and 98 years were cobalamin deficient.[1] A study in Georgia in 2010 evaluated the prevalence of B12 deficiency (defined as <258 pmol/L) in patients of various ethnic background aged 80 to 89 and greater than 98 years. Among this geriatric population not receiving vitamin B12 replacement, the centenarians were found to have a higher prevalence of B12 deficiency at 35% versus 23% among octogenarians.[9] The KORA-Age study evaluated 1079 residents in the city of Augsburg, Germany and found that 27% of participants (aged 65–93 years) demonstrated laboratory evidence of vitamin B12 deficiency (defined as <221 pmol/L). The prevalence of B12 deficiency among those participants aged 85 to 93 years was significantly higher, at 38%.[10]

The mechanism accounting for anemia in community-dwelling elderly (those 65 years and older) was examined by Guralnik and associates from data derived in the NHANES III study.[11] In that large dataset, 11% met the WHO criteria for anemia (hemoglobin <12 g/dL for women and <13 g/dL for men). Of these, iron deficiency accounted for 16.6%, whereas B12 deficiency accounted for 5.9%. The combination of folic acid and B12 deficiency added another 2%. Unexplained anemia (See William B. Ershler's article, "Unexplained Anemia in the Elderly," in this issue) accounted for approximately one-third of the observed anemia in the population sampled.

CLINICAL MANIFESTATIONS

The clinical presentation of vitamin B12 deficiency is manifold but primarily presents with neurologic or hematologic abnormalities. The hematologic manifestations can be diverse, including leukopenia, anemia, and thrombocytopenia. The neurologic manifestations often present as distal peripheral neuropathy but can be as severe as subacute combined degeneration of the dorsal columns or cerebellar symptoms.[1] Less common manifestations include glossitis, atrophy of the skin, or seemingly unrelated symptoms such as dementia and venous thrombosis due to hyperhomocysteinemia.[5,12,13]

Adding to the subtlety of the diagnosis, consideration of B12 deficiency in patients who present without anemia is important. For example, Healton and colleagues[14] found that 21% of the 147 B12-deficient patients who had been referred for neurologic symptoms over a 17-year period were not anemic. In another observational cohort that included 201 patients evaluated at a single institution, nearly half reported neurologic or psychiatric symptoms at the time of diagnosis and 28% had no hematologic abnormalities.[15]

Furthermore, a recent study of 165 Taiwanese patients, median age 76 years, with mild to moderate Alzheimer dementia on cholinesterase inhibitors found an inverse correlation between vitamin B12 levels and progression of dementia.[12] It is hypothesized that vitamin B12 may play a role in dementia as deficiencies are associated with a loss of white matter of the brain and spinal cord. One theory suggests that insufficient B12 leads to defective methylation of myelin basic protein.[12] However, supplementation of vitamin B12 has not yet demonstrated improvement in Alzheimer dementia.[16]

DIAGNOSIS

The evaluation of vitamin B12 deficiency begins with testing a serum vitamin B12 level. Macrocytic anemia supports a suspected diagnosis of B12 deficiency, although it is not essential, as mentioned earlier. Typically, the mean corpuscular volume begins to increase once the vitamin B12 level is <200 ng/L.[3] By contrast, MMA and homocysteine levels are both more sensitive and specific for the diagnosis of B12 deficiency.[3] A Mayo Clinic series of 72 patients found increased MMA levels in a patient with a B12 level of 400 ng/L (295 pmol/L).[3]

According to the study of Andrès and colleagues,[1] the definition of cobalamin deficiency is a serum cobalamin level less than 150 pmol/L on 2 separate occasions or a serum cobalamin level less than 150 pmol/L and a total serum homocysteine level greater than 13 μmol/L, or a methylmalonic acid greater than 0.4 μmol/mL, in the absence of renal failure or folate and B12 deficiency. However, as pointed out by Solomon,[17] there is considerable uncertainty about the diagnostic criteria and probably no single laboratory value is sufficient.

Of note, there is some evidence to suggest that significantly increased titers of intrinsic factor antibodies may result in falsely normal serum cobalamin levels.[18] Therefore, a high index of suspicion should prompt additional testing for vitamin B12 deficiency despite an apparently normal serum level. In addition, there are conditions that have been associated with falsely low B12 levels, including folate deficiency, pregnancy, and transcobalamin deficiencies; these should be considered when diagnosing true deficiency.[3,19]

There is a third assay, the holotranscobalamin, that is more sensitive than a serum vitamin B12 level. In contrast to the serum vitamin B12 assay, which evaluates the combined active and inactive forms of vitamin B12, the holotranscobalamin evaluates the active portion of the vitamin.[19]

ETIOLOGY

There are multiple causes of vitamin B12 deficiency to be considered. Mild B12 deficiency is often caused by drugs that interrupt the normal absorption of vitamin B12, such as metformin, H2 inhibitors, and proton pump inhibitors.[1,2] Of note there is some controversy as to whether metformin results in actual vitamin B12 deficiency or only a low serum vitamin B12 level while not affecting intracellular vitamin B12 levels.[20,21] Similarly, vegan diets may result in vitamin B12 deficiency, although it typically takes several years of compliance with a vegan diet for this to manifest. A more severe B12 deficiency is observed when there is an inability to absorb B12, such as in pernicious anemia or gastrectomy, in which the production of intrinsic factor is diminished, or ileal resection,[2] in which the distal absorption of B12 is affected. Rarer causes of B12 deficiency include inflammatory diseases of the ileum, pancreatic exocrine deficiency, and *Diphyllobothrium latum* parasitic infection.[1]

In particular, the elderly seem to be at higher risk for pernicious anemia and food cobalamin malabsorption.[1,22] Food cobalamin malabsorption is characterized by the inability to release cobalamin from food or from intestinal transport proteins, particularly in the presence of hypochlorhydria. This syndrome is defined by the presence of cobalamin deficiency despite adequate dietary intake. In this type of malabsorption, the Schilling test,[23] which uses the oral administration of crystallized vitamin B12, will be normal. The cause of food cobalamin malabsorption is predominantly gastric atrophy, which is far more prominent in the elderly. Over 40% of patients who are more than 80 years of age have gastric atrophy, which may or may not be related to *Helicobacter pylori* infection.[1] The causes of B12 deficiency in the elderly (and the approximate frequency with which they occur) are shown in **Box 1**. Other factors that contribute to food cobalamin malabsorption are shown in **Box 2**.

CLINICAL APPLICATION AND TREATMENT

The British Committee for Standards in Hematology has incorporated the aforementioned data into an algorithmic format to assist the practitioner with specific guidelines for the workup and treatment of vitamin B12 deficiency. If a vitamin B12 level is checked for nonspecific symptoms (ie, without clear evidence of neuropathy, glossitis, or anemia), and without significant laboratory abnormalities and results <150 ng/L (110 pmol/L), the patient should undergo investigation and treatment for presumed pernicious anemia. However, if the vitamin B12 level results between 150 and 200 ng/L (110–148 pmol/L) it is reasonable repeat the measure in 1 to 2 months, because the repeated measure is frequently within the normal range, and, under those circumstances, no additional evaluation is recommended. However, if the repeat vitamin B12 level remains less than 200 ng/L, empiric therapy can be considered and subsequent investigation for pernicious anemia with an intrinsic factor antibody is warranted. If the intrinsic factor antibody is negative, the serum vitamin B12 should be evaluated for a third time. If it is more than 200 ng/L, no further investigation is required. However, if the serum B12 level remains between 150 and 200 ng/L the deficiency should be confirmed with MMA, homocysteine, or holotranscobalamin levels. If the deficiency is confirmed with these laboratory tests it is reasonable to consider treatment for antibody-negative pernicious anemia.[19]

By contrast, these same guidelines recommend that all patients with symptoms correlating with a high clinical suspicion (ie, glossitis or neuropathy) or objective laboratory evidence of vitamin B12 deficiency (anemia) and a serum B12 level less

---

Box 1
Causes of B12 deficiency in older patients

- Food cobalamin malabsorption (60%–70%)
- Pernicious anemia (15%–20%)
- Dietary deficiency (<5%)
- Malabsorption (<5%)
- Hereditary causes (<1%)

Data from Andres E, Loukili NH, Noel E, et al. Vitamin B12 (cobalamin) deficiency in elderly patients. CMAJ 2004;171(3):251–9.

Box 2
Other factors that contribute to malabsorption of vitamin B12 in older people.

- Intestinal microbial proliferation
- Chronic alcoholism
- Gastric reconstruction
- Pancreatic enzyme deficiency
- Sjogren syndrome
- Long-term ingestion of drugs
  - Biguanides
  - Antacids
  - H2 receptor antagonists
  - Proton pump inhibitors

Data from Andres E, Loukili NH, Noel E, et al. Vitamin B12 (cobalamin) deficiency in elderly patients. CMAJ 2004;171(3):251–9.

---

than 200 ng/L undergo further evaluation for pernicious anemia and begin empiric therapy while these laboratory tests are pending. If, however, a patient has a serum B12 level greater than 200 ng/L, but B12 deficiency is still suspected (given the prevalence of falsely increased serum B12 levels), the suspected diagnosis and cause should be further investigated with a serum MMA, homocysteine, holotranscobalamin level, and intrinsic factor antibody. While these results are pending, empiric therapy should be initiated.[19]

The treatment of vitamin B12 deficiency depends on the cause of the deficiency. For patients with pernicious anemia due to impaired intrinsic factor function or neurologic symptoms, parenteral supplementation with cobalamin injections (1000 μg) several times per week for 1 to 2 weeks, followed by weekly injections for 1 month, is recommended.[2,19,24] A maintenance dose is then provided varying from monthly to bimonthly[2] for patients with neurologic symptoms on presentation, to quarterly for those without initial neurologic symptoms.[19] Interestingly, there is evidence to suggest that oral supplementation is still effective in patients with impaired intrinsic factor function or loss of the terminal ileum when sufficiently high doses of vitamin B12 are provided due to passive diffusion across mucus membranes.[2,19,24–26] In elderly patients, in whom impaired gastric absorption seems to be a predominant cause of vitamin B12 deficiency,[27] oral supplementation at very high doses has been found to be effective at reducing MMA levels. A dose finding trial by Eussen[28] found that daily oral doses of 500 μg were required to lower MMA levels by 33%. Similarly, Andrès and colleagues[22] found that oral vitamin B12 supplementation in 10 patients produced an improvement in vitamin B12 levels and hematologic parameters in most patients treated with 5000 μg of oral vitamin B12 weekly. However, given concerns regarding compliance in the elderly, parenteral administration may be a more effective means to ensure adequate repletion.

SUMMARY

Vitamin B12 deficiency exists at a fairly high prevalence in the elderly population. As the general population ages, clinicians need to be aware of the myriad of ways in which vitamin B12 can present. These can often be iatrogenic (such as polypharmacy and bariatric surgery), autoimmune, or as yet unclear, as in the case of gastric atrophy and its possible association with *H. pylori*. Furthermore, it is essential to properly investigate the suspected cause of vitamin B12 deficiency, because the type and duration of treatment varies. In elderly patients, clinicians should maintain a high index of suspicion that vitamin B12 deficiency may be the cause of, or contributing to, commonly observed vague symptoms (eg, fatigue, paresthesias, mild gait abnormalities). This is particularly salient given the fairly high prevalence of vitamin B12 deficiency and the relative ease of treatment. In particular, clinicians should be aware of the high prevalence of food cobalamin malabsorption as a common cause, and become comfortable initiating appropriate patient-centered treatment most likely to produce clinical response.

REFERENCES

1. Andres E, Loukili NH, Noel E, et al. Vitamin B12 (cobalamin) deficiency in elderly patients. CMAJ 2004;171(3):251–9.
2. Green R. Vitamin B12 deficiency from the perspective of a practicing hematologist. Blood 2017;129(19):2603–11.
3. Klee GG. Cobalamin and folate evaluation: measurement of methylmalonic acid and homocysteine vs vitamin B(12) and folate. Clin Chem 2000;46(8 Pt 2): 1277–83.
4. Institute of Medicine. Dietary reference intakes for thiamin, riboflavin, niacin, vitamin B6, folate, vitamin B12, pantothenic acid, biotin and choline. Washington (DC): National Academy Press; 1998.
5. Andres E, Noel E, Kaltenbach G, et al. Vitamin B12 deficiency with normal Schilling test or non-dissociation of vitamin B12 and its carrier proteins in elderly patients. A study of 60 patients. Rev Med Interne 2003;24(4):218–23 [in French].
6. Andres E, Perrin AE, Demangeat C, et al. The syndrome of food-cobalamin malabsorption revisited in a department of internal medicine. A monocentric cohort study of 80 patients. Eur J Intern Med 2003;14(4):221–6.
7. Lindenbaum J, Rosenberg IH, Wilson PW, et al. Prevalence of cobalamin deficiency in the Framingham elderly population. Am J Clin Nutr 1994;60(1):2–11.
8. van Asselt DZ, Blom HJ, Zuiderent R, et al. Clinical significance of low cobalamin levels in older hospital patients. Neth J Med 2000;57(2):41–9.
9. Johnson MA, Hausman DB, Davey A, et al. Vitamin B12 deficiency in African American and white octogenarians and centenarians in Georgia. J Nutr Health Aging 2010;14(5):339–45.
10. Conzade R, Koenig W, Heier M, et al. Prevalence and predictors of subclinical micronutrient deficiency in German older adults: results from the population-based KORA-age study. Nutrients 2017;9(12) [pii:E1276].
11. Guralnik JM, Eisenstaedt RS, Ferrucci L, et al. Prevalence of anemia in persons 65 years and older in the United States: evidence for a high rate of unexplained anemia. Blood 2004;104(8):2263–8.
12. Cho HS, Huang LK, Lee YT, et al. Suboptimal baseline serum vitamin B12 is associated with cognitive decline in people with Alzheimer's disease undergoing cholinesterase inhibitor treatment. Front Neurol 2018;9:325.
13. den Heijer M, Koster T, Blom HJ, et al. Hyperhomocysteinemia as a risk factor for deep-vein thrombosis. N Engl J Med 1996;334(12):759–62.
14. Healton EB, Savage DG, Brust JC, et al. Neurologic aspects of cobalamin deficiency. Medicine (Baltimore) 1991;70(4):229–45.

15. Andres E, Affenberger S, Zimmer J, et al. Current hematological findings in cobalamin deficiency. A study of 201 consecutive patients with documented cobalamin deficiency. Clin Lab Haematol 2006;28(1):50–6.
16. Zhang DM, Ye JX, Mu JS, et al. Efficacy of vitamin B supplementation on cognition in elderly patients with cognitive-related diseases. J Geriatr Psychiatry Neurol 2017;30(1):50–9.
17. Solomon LR. Cobalamin-responsive disorders in the ambulatory care setting: unreliability of cobalamin, methylmalonic acid, and homocysteine testing. Blood 2005;105(3):978–85 [author reply: 1137].
18. Hamilton MS, Blackmore S, Lee A. Possible cause of false normal B-12 assays. BMJ 2006;333(7569):654–5.
19. Devalia V, Hamilton MS, Molloy AM, et al. Guidelines for the diagnosis and treatment of cobalamin and folate disorders. Br J Haematol 2014;166(4):496–513.
20. Obeid R. Metformin causing vitamin B12 deficiency: a guilty verdict without sufficient evidence. Diabetes Care 2014;37(2):e22–3.
21. Sugrue A, Egan A, Oregan A. A woman with macrocytic anaemia and confusion. BMJ 2014;349:g4388.
22. Andrès E, Kurtz J-E, Perrin A-E, et al. Oral cobalamin therapy for the treatment of patients with food-cobalamin malabsorption. Am J Med 2001;111(2):126–9.
23. Abels J, Schilling RF. Protection of intrinsic factor by vitamin B12. J Lab Clin Med 1964;64:375–84.
24. Stabler S. Vitamin B12 deficiency. N Engl J Med 2013;368(2):149–60.
25. Berlin H, Berlin R, Brante G. Oral treatment of pernicious anemia with high doses of vitamin B12 without intrinsic factor. Acta Med Scand 1968;184:247–58.
26. Vidal-Alaball J, Butler C, Cannings-John R, et al. Oral vitamin B12 versus intramuscular vitamin B12 for vitamin B12 deficiency. Cochrane Database Syst Rev 2005;(3):CD004655.
27. Andrès E, Perrin A, Kraemer J, et al. Anemia caused by vitamin B12 deficiency in elderly subjects over 75 years of age: new hypotheses and a study of 20 cases. Rev Med Interne 2000;21(11):946–54.
28. Eussen SJPM. Oral cyanocobalamin supplementation in older people with vitamin B12 deficiency. Arch Intern Med 2005;165(10):1167.

Kidney Disease and Anemia in Elderly Patients

Franco Musio, MD[a,b],*

KEYWORDS

- Anemia • Elderly • Chronic kidney disease • Erythroid stimulating agents

KEY POINTS

- Various equations are available for the assessment of renal function in the elderly to include the Cockcroft–Gault, Modification of Diet in Renal Disease, and CKD-EPI equations, although they tend to underestimate the true glomerular filtration rate (GFR).
- The prevalence and severity of anemia increase as GFR becomes less than 60 mL/min due to impaired synthesis of erythropoietin, although iron deficiency, chronic inflammation, and malnutrition may also contribute.
- Anemia in the elderly is associated with increased risk for cardiovascular and cerebrovascular disease, hospitalization, functional decline, reduced quality of life, and mortality.
- Although opinions vary as to the optimal target hemoglobin level in the setting of erythropoetin therapy, elderly patients with chronic kidney disease should be treated.

INTRODUCTION

Anemia is a well-known complicating feature of chronic kidney disease (CKD) and typically correlates directly with the degree of kidney impairment (**Table 1**). The operational diagnosis of anemia in the elderly is a matter of some debate.[1–3] Further, the optimal measure of kidney function in the elderly is yet to be established.

The association of CKD and anemia has been thoroughly reviewed elsewhere,[4,5] and this report focuses on topics particularly relevant to geriatric population with emphasis on the assessment of kidney function in the elderly, the diagnosis and impact of CKD-related anemia in the elderly, and treatment of elderly patients with CKD-related anemia.

Disclosure Statement: The author has nothing to disclose.
[a] Nephrology Section, Department of Medicine, Inova Fairfax Hospital, Annandale, VA, USA;
[b] Nephrology Associates of Northern Virginia, 13135 Lee Jackson Memorial Highway, Suite 135, Fairfax, VA 22033, USA
* Nephrology Associates of Northern Virginia, 13135 Lee Jackson Memorial Highway, Suite 135, Fairfax, VA 22033.
E-mail address: Franco.Musio@inova.org

Clin Geriatr Med 35 (2019) 327–337
https://doi.org/10.1016/j.cger.2019.03.009
0749-0690/19/© 2019 Elsevier Inc. All rights reserved.

geriatric.theclinics.com

Table 1 Stages of chronic kidney disease		
Stage	Description	GFR (mL/min/ 1.73 m^2)
1	Kidney damage with normal or increased GFR	≥90
2	Kidney damage with mild decrease in GFR	60–89
3	Moderate decrease in GFR	30–59
4	Severe decrease in GFR	15–29
5	Kidney failure	<15 (or dialysis)

Abbreviation: GFR, glomerular filtration rate.

ASSESSMENT OF KIDNEY FUNCTION IN THE ELDERLY

Kidney function commonly declines with age, although not universally.[6–9] Approximately one-third of elderly adults do not exhibit an age-related decline in kidney function.[7] This has led to the suggestion that a decline in GFR is not a normal accompaniment of aging *per se*, but rather due to the coexistence of hypertension, cardiovascular disease, and/or diabetes mellitus. By the age of 80 years, mean GFR, depending on how it is measured or estimated, is approximately 50 to 80 mL/min, compared with 120 mL/min or greater in individuals in their 20s to 40s. Despite this reduced level of glomerular filtration rate (GFR) with advanced age, serum creatinine levels tend to remain relatively unchanged or increase only modestly over time in the absence of chronic disease. This is thought to be secondary to reduced muscle mass (sarcopenia) that often accompanies aging.[7,10–12]

Kidney function is typically assessed by measurement of serum creatinine, collection of a 24-hour urine for creatinine clearance, or use of the Cockcroft–Gault equation[13] to estimate GFR. In the elderly, reduction in muscle mass, compared with younger subjects, distorts the relationship between serum creatinine and estimated GFR (eGFR) using the Cockcroft–Gault formula so that serum creatinine typically underestimates the severity of CKD.

Recent developments have greatly improved the clinical evaluation of kidney function. First, as the result of the analysis of a wealth of data from the Modification of Diet in Renal Disease (MDRD) Study, prediction equations have been derived that can more precisely provide an eGFR.[14] Although still imperfect, use of the so-called abbreviated or modified MDRD prediction equation has increasingly gained acceptance as an important clinical tool for assessing GFR.

The Cockcroft–Gault formula was derived over 40 years ago from 236 hospitalized men between the ages of 18 and 92 years.[13] Several MDRD equations, with the 4-variable version being most popular, were derived and validated in 1628 subjects (mean age of 50.6 years) with precise GFR measurements and laboratory data,[14] thus their generalizability to older subjects was initially unclear (**Table 2**). More recently the CKD-EPI equation has been developed and is considered to be equivalent to the MDRD for patients with CKD and more accurate for individuals with eGFR greater than 60 mL/min.[15] Investigators have recently evaluated the Cockcroft–Gault, MDRD, and CDK-EPI equations with a focus on the elderly.[16,17] They found a fairly good correlation, although it is notable that the Cockcroft–Gault formula tended to systematically underestimate GFR.[6]

Verhave and colleagues compared the Cockcroft–Gault formula and modified MDRD equation (using serum creatinine, gender, and age) with 99mTc-DTPA renal clearance measurements in 850 subjects. Among those 65 years or older, both the

Table 2						
Serum creatinine concentrations corresponding to eGFR levels of 60 mL/min/1.73 m² by the abbreviated MDRD equation or 60 mL/min by the Cockcroft–Gault equation						
	MDRD Equation				Cockcroft–Gault	
	European-American		African-American			
Age (yrs)	Men	Women	Men	Women	Men	Women
50	1.34	1.03	1.58	1.22	1.50	1.28
60	1.30	1.00	1.53	1.18	1.33	1.13
70	1.26	0.97	1.49	1.15	1.17	0.99
80	1.23	0.95	1.46	1.12	1.00	0.85

Calculations assume weight of 72 kg and body surface area of 1.73 m². Creatinine in mg/dL.
Adapted from Levey AS, Bosch JP, Lewis JB, et al. A more accurate method to estimate glomerular filtration rate from serum creatinine: a new prediction equation. Modification of Diet in Renal Disease Study Group. Ann Intern Med 1999;130(6):461–70; with permission.

Cockcroft–Gault and the MDRD formulas underestimated GFR, with the underestimation greater for the Cockcroft-Gault formula.[18] Similar observations of underestimation of GFR by Cockcroft Gault equation compared with MDRD have been reported by other investigators.[19,20]

ANEMIA DUE TO CHRONIC KIDNEY DISEASE IN THE ELDERLY

A normochromic normocytic anemia is a well-known complication of CKD.[5,21] Findings from the NHANES III study (in which the mean age was 48 years) indicate that hemoglobin levels typically begin to decline as the GFR becomes less than 70 mL/min in men and 50 mL/min in women and that the prevalence and severity of anemia increase as kidney function becomes less than a level of about 60 mL/min. The prevalence of hemoglobin levels less than 11 g/dL increases as GFR becomes less than about 30 mL/min/ 1.73 m².[5,14,22–24] The principal underlying cause of CKD-related anemia is impaired synthesis of the glycoprotein hormone erythropoietin, which is produced primarily by the cortical fibroblasts adjacent to the peritubular capillaries of the proximal convoluted tubules. Other important contributing factors include iron deficiency, chronic inflammation, and malnutrition, each of which is more likely to occur in the elderly.[25]

Among community dwelling individuals older than the age of 65 years, CKD is the most common causes of anemia.[22] The pathophysiologic basis for anemia related to CKD in older individuals is likely similar to that of younger subjects, complicated perhaps by a greater impact of underlying inflammatory processes, and in men, an age-related decline in testosterone levels.[23,24] Data from the Baltimore Longitudinal Study on Aging (BLSA) revealed an increase in serum erythropoietin level with advancing age with or without the occurrence of anemia.[26,27] Notably, in the BLSA study[26] the increase in erythropoietin levels was less marked in subjects with hypertension or diabetes mellitus, perhaps reflecting some underlying CKD, either age-related or due to these other conditions. Although some studies suggest that the erythropoietin production in response to anemia and erythropoietin responsiveness is blunted in healthy elderly subjects, others have found no difference comparing older and younger subjects and most have not considered the effect of underlying CKD.[26–34]

One assessment of the association of anemia and CKD in the elderly comes from the InCHIANTI study, a prospective, population-based survey of older residents of

Tuscany, Italy, who were at least 65 years old (mean 74.5 years; range 65–102 years) and in whom anemia was defined using the WHO criteria (hemoglobin <12 g/dL in women and <13 g/dL in men).[35] In both men and women, the prevalence of anemia was greater at older ages and both hemoglobin and 24-hour creatinine clearance declined with increasing age. The mean age-related decline in hemoglobin and creatinine clearance was 0.75 g/dL and 19.4 mL/min per decade, respectively, in men and 0.50 g/dL and 15.2 mL/min per decade, respectively, in women. The unadjusted prevalence of anemia, using WHO criteria, was higher among men and women at lower levels of creatinine clearance, particularly among subjects with creatinine clearance of 60 mL/min or less. The prevalence was 6.6% in subjects with creatinine clearance greater than 90%, 9.8% in those with creatinine clearance of 61 to 90 mL/min, 18.5% among those with creatinine clearance of 31 to 60 mL/min, and 65.4% in those with creatinine clearance of 30 mL/min or less. In age- and sex-adjusted comparisons, the prevalence of anemia was greater only in the group with creatinine clearance levels of 30 mL/min or less. Serum erythropoietin levels declined with lower levels of kidney function. Age and hemoglobin-adjusted levels were significantly lower only in subjects with creatinine clearance of 30 mL/min or less, compared with the group with creatinine clearance greater than 90 mL/min. The authors of this study concluded that among older individuals, the age-related decline in erythropoietin synthesis was an important contributing factor to anemia only when kidney function was severely impaired, that is, when creatinine clearance was 30 mL/min or less.

In an earlier study of subjects between the ages of 49 and 97 years, there was also an inverse relationship between creatinine clearance (estimated with the Cockcroft–Gault formula) and prevalence of anemia (using WHO criteria), with a greater than 5-fold risk of anemia among men and greater than 3-fold risk of anemia in women with creatinine clearance less than 50 mL/min compared with those with higher creatinine clearance.[10] In the entire study population, it was estimated that in approximately 17% of women and 22% of men, anemia could be attributed to renal impairment.

EFFECTS OF ANEMIA ON ELDERLY PATIENTS WITH CHRONIC KIDNEY DISEASE

In the general elderly, and particularly in the frail elderly with CKD, anemia has clearly been associated with reduced quality of life (QOL), increased hospitalization risk, longer hospital stays, functional decline, greater cardiovascular and cerebrovascular disease burden, and increased mortality.[36] Less is known of the anemia-related impact specifically among elderly subjects with CKD. In a study of more than 17,000 residents of Calgary, Canada, who were 66 years of age or older,[37] anemia was associated with a 5-fold increase in the risk for all-cause mortality in an adjusted analysis. When assessed in terms of baseline GFR, the hazard ratio for mortality risk associated with anemia in subjects with a normal GFR was 4.29, compared with 2.80 in subjects with a GFR of 30 to 59 mL/min/1.73 m², and 1.53 in those with a GFR less than 30 mL/min/1.73 m². Thus, the incremental risk of death associated with anemia was actually greater at higher levels of kidney function than at lower levels, although in both anemic and nonanemic subjects, lower levels of GFR were associated with higher mortality.

In a retrospective study of a representative Medicare database, in patients aged 67 years or older anemia was associated with increased risk of atherosclerotic vascular disease, congestive heart failure, renal replacement therapy, and death.[38] Anemia may also be a risk factor for cognitive impairment associated with CKD in the elderly.[39]

Using analysis of approximately 6 years of medical and pharmacy claims from a large managed care database, Lefebvre and colleagues[40] assessed costs associated with untreated anemia in subjects 65 years of age or older with eGFR less than 60 mL/min/1.73 m². Observation periods with and without anemia were compared. Untreated anemia was associated with a significant increase in health care costs; compared to periods of time when anemia was not present, monthly costs for outpatient services, inpatient services, and total costs were 1.4- to 2-fold higher. Inpatient services were the most significant factor associated with higher costs in anemic compared with non-anemic periods. Pharmacy costs were not higher during periods of untreated anemia. In multivariate analysis, it was determined that the cost burden of anemia in these older subjects was comparable to those associated with diabetes, coronary artery disease, and other comorbidities. The lower the hemoglobin level and GFR, the higher the overall costs of care.

TREATMENT OF ANEMIA IN ELDERLY PATIENTS WITH CHRONIC KIDNEY DISEASE

Recombinant human erythropoietin (epoetin) therapy revolutionized the treatment of anemia for both patients with end-stage renal disease on dialysis or for those with CKD not receiving dialysis.[4,41,42] Various alterations to the erythropoietin molecule have been engineered to provide more desirable pharmacokinetics[43–46] and still others are in development.[47] Although, as a group erythroid-stimulating agents (ESAs) have proved quite safe, there were early concerns raised about the possibility of enhanced tumor proliferative properties causing US Food and Drug Administration (FDA) warnings and more restricted use in patients with cancer.[48] Furthermore, the specific risks and benefits, as well as costs, of such treatment in the elderly with or without CKD have not been well characterized.

Among elderly subjects with no CKD, responsiveness to exogenous epoetin does not seem to be impaired when compared with younger subjects.[30,49] Also, limited data suggest that epoetin responsiveness in older hemodialysis patients is similar to younger hemodialysis patients.[50] Despite similar monthly epoetin doses, the mean monthly hemoglobin level among dialysis patients 75 years and older tend to be lower than younger patients. Among elderly hemodialysis patients, the impact of epoetin therapy on QOL has been mixed. Although one small study questioned the benefit,[51] a larger, controlled trial found that the improvements in QOL scores after 6 month of epoetin treatment were of similar magnitude in hemodialysis patients 60 years of age and older compared with those less than 60 years, although absolute QOL scores were lower both before and after treatment in the older subjects.[52]

Given the limited data available, elderly patients with CKD, whether on dialysis or not, should probably be evaluated and treated for their anemia as generally recommended for younger patients with CKD.[5] The most recent clinical practice guidelines and recommendations for the National Kidney Foundation Kidney Disease Outcome Quality Initiative (KDOQI) for Anemia in CKD recommend that hemoglobin testing be carried out at least annually in all patients with CKD, regardless of stage or cause, and that a diagnosis of anemia should be made and evaluation should be undertaken when the hemoglobin level is less than 13.5 g/dL in adult men and 12.0 g/dL in adult women. This evaluation should include a complete blood count, red blood cell indices (mean corpuscular hemoglobin, mean corpuscular volume, mean corpuscular hemoglobin concentration), white blood cell count, differential and platelet count, absolute reticulocyte count, serum ferritin to assess iron stores, and serum TSAT or content of hemoglobin in reticulocytes to assess adequacy of iron for erythropoiesis. Among patients treated with ESA therapy and/or iron, the initial 2006 guidelines recommended a lower limit of hemoglobin in patients with CKD at 11.0 g/dL.[5] In the opinion of the KDOQI Anemia Work Group, there was insufficient evidence to recommend routinely maintaining hemoglobin levels at 13.0 g/dL or greater in ESA-treated patients. Since adequate iron stores are essential for optimal erythropoiesis, with or without ESA therapy, the Anemia Work Group recommended that sufficient iron be administered to maintain the serum ferritin concentration greater than 200 ng/mL in hemodialysis patients and greater than 100 ng/mL in CKD patients not on dialysis and those on peritoneal dialysis, with a TSAT greater than 20% in all patients. In addition, in the opinion of the Work Group, there was insufficient evidence to recommend routine administration of intravenous (IV) iron if serum ferritin level is greater than 500 ng/mL. When ferritin level is greater than 500 ng/mL, decisions regarding IV iron administration need to consider ESA responsiveness, hemoglobin levels over time, the TSAT level, and the patient's clinical status.

An early clinical trial report resulted in a recalibration of target hemoglobin to levels lower than 13 g/dL. This was a randomized controlled trial in hemodialysis patients that compared a target hematocrit level of 30% versus 42%. The trial was terminated early when it became apparent that there was no benefit in patients assigned to the higher hematocrit target.[53] The risk of the primary composite outcome of first nonfatal myocardial infarction or death was 30% higher in the normal hematocrit group than the low hematocrit group, although this was not statistically significantly different when the study was stopped. The incidence of thrombosis of vascular access sites was higher in the normal hematocrit group than in the low hematocrit group. There were no differences in the rates of occurrence for all-cause hospitalization for all causes, nonfatal myocardial infarction, angina pectoris requiring hospitalization, congestive heart failure requiring hospitalization, coronary-artery bypass grafting, or percutaneous transluminal coronary angioplasty.

Similarly, a large randomized controlled trial in patients with CKD not on dialysis was also terminated early, with a significantly higher rate of composite events (death, myocardial infarction, hospitalization for congestive heart failure without renal replacement therapy, and stroke) among subjects randomized to a target hemoglobin level of 13.0 to 13.5 g/dL compared with those randomized to a target hemoglobin level of 10.5 to 11.0 g/dL (a later protocol amendment changed the targets to 13.5 g/dL and 11.3 g/dL, respectively).[54] A mean hemoglobin level of 12.6 g/dL was achieved in the higher target group. The risk for the single outcome events of death and congestive heart failure hospitalization approached being statistically significantly greater ($P = .07$) in the higher hemoglobin group. Other studies have also shown either no benefit or a significant trend toward increased risk for some outcomes when hemoglobin levels are normalized with ESA therapy in patients with CKD.[55–57] Lastly, current KDOQI guidelines have included additional randomized controlled trials since the 2006 practice guidelines. In the opinion of the Anemia Work Group, the recommended hemoglobin target in dialysis and nondialysis patients with CKD is in the range of 11.0 to 12.0 g/dL. The 2012 Kidney Disease: Improving Global Outcomes (KDIGO) Clinical Practice Guidelines for Anemia in CKD recommendations include an upper target hemoglobin level of 11.5 g/dL.[58] Provision was made for individualization of therapy for targets above 11.5 g/dL to improve QOL, although potential risks would need to be accepted by the patient. The most recent KDOQI recommendations come as a response to the above KDIGO guidelines. As a KDOQI US Commentary, the Anemia Group endorses the FDA upper limit of 11.0 g/dL at which point ESA therapy should be interrupted.[59]

In summary, until further analysis and information become available, most ESA-treated patients with CKD should have their hemoglobin levels maintained greater

Table 3
Key ESA trials in patients with chronic kidney disease

	Normal Hematocrit Study (NHS) (N = 1265)[53]	CHOIR (N = 1432)[54]	TREAT (N = 4038)[61]
Time Period of Trial	1993–1996	2003–2006	2004–2009
Population	Patients with CKD on hemodialysis with coexisting CHF or CAD, hematocrit 30 ± 3% on epoetin alfa	Patients with CKD not on dialysis with hemoglobin <11 g/dL not previously administered epoetin alfa	Patients with CKD not on dialysis with type II diabetes, hemoglobin ≤11 g/dL
Hemoglobin Target; Higher vs Lower (g/dL)	14.0 vs 10.0	13.5 vs 11.3	13.0 vs ≥9.0
Median (Q1, Q3) Achieved Hemoglobin Level (g/dL)	12.6 (11.6, 13.3) vs 10.3 (10.0, 10.7)	13.0 (12.2, 13.4) vs 11.4 (11.1, 11.6)	12.5 (12.0, 12.8) vs 10.6 (9.9, 11.3)
Primary Endpoint	All-cause mortality or nonfatal MI	All-cause mortality, MI, hospitalization for CHF, or stroke	All-cause mortality, MI, myocardial ischemia, heart failure, and stroke
Hazard Ratio or Relative Risk (95% CI)	1.28 (1.06–1.56)	1.34 (1.03–1.74)	1.05 (0.94–1.17)
Adverse Outcome for Higher Target Group	All-cause mortality	All-cause mortality	Stroke
Hazard Ratio or Relative Risk (95% CI)	1.27 (1.04–1.54)	1.48 (0.97–2.27)	1.92 (1.38–2.68)

Abbreviations: CAD, coronary artery disease; CHF, congestive heart failure; CHOIR, correction of hemoglobin and outcomes in renal insufficiency trial; CI, confidence interval; MI, myocardial infarction; TREAT, trial to reduce cardiovascular events with Aranesp therapy.

From FDA. Drug safety communication: modified dosing recommendations to improve the safe use of erythropoiesis-stimulating agents (ESAs) in chronic kidney disease. Available at: https://www.fda.gov/Drugs/DrugSafety/ucm259639.htm. Accessed January 21, 2019.

than 11.0 g/dL but less than 13.0 g/dL and perhaps even lower. In fact, a recent FDA alert, issued after the 2 CKD reports,[54,55] advised adherence to prescribing information for currently available ESAs, recommending the target hemoglobin be maintained at 10 g/dL (**Table 3**).[60]

SUMMARY

Anemia and CKD are both common underrecognized and undertreated conditions with significant effects on morbidity and mortality in the elderly. Recognizing the presence of CKD by determination of eGFR rather than relying on whether a serum creatinine concentration is "normal" or not is of paramount importance in the elderly. Elderly patients with CKD and anemia should have a thorough evaluation for causes other than, or in addition to, their CKD; often iron deficiency or other conditions to include inflammatory insults will be found to be present. Once these other treatable conditions are corrected, appropriate therapy with epoetin or other ESAs should be offered when appropriate, adhering to recommended treatment and monitoring guidelines.

REFERENCES

1. Chaves PH, Xue QL, Guralnik JM, et al. What constitutes normal hemoglobin concentration in community-dwelling disabled older women? J Am Geriatr Soc 2004; 52(11):1811–6.
2. Izaks GJ, Westendorp RG, Knook DL. The definition of anemia in older persons. JAMA 1999;281(18):1714–7.
3. Semba RD, Ricks MO, Ferrucci L, et al. Types of anemia and mortality among older disabled women living in the community: the Women's Health and Aging Study I. Aging Clin Exp Res 2007;19(4):259–64.
4. Eschbach JW. The anemia of chronic renal failure: pathophysiology and the effects of recombinant erythropoietin. Kidney Int 1989;35(1):134–48.
5. KDOQI, National Kidney Foundation. KDOQI clinical practice guidelines and clinical practice recommendations for anemia in chronic kidney disease. Am J Kidney Dis 2006;47(5 Suppl 3):S11–145.
6. Fehrman-Ekholm I, Skeppholm L. Renal function in the elderly (>70 years old) measured by means of iohexol clearance, serum creatinine, serum urea and estimated clearance. Scand J Urol Nephrol 2004;38(1):73–7.
7. Lindeman RD, Tobin J, Shock NW. Longitudinal studies on the rate of decline in renal function with age. J Am Geriatr Soc 1985;33(4):278–85.
8. Nicoll SR, Sainsbury R, Bailey RR, et al. Assessment of creatinine clearance in healthy subjects over 65 years of age. Nephron 1991;59(4):621–5.
9. Rowe JW, Andres R, Tobin JD, et al. The effect of age on creatinine clearance in men: a cross-sectional and longitudinal study. J Gerontol 1976;31(2):155–63.
10. Cumming RG, Mitchell P, Craig JC, et al. Renal impairment and anaemia in a population-based study of older people. Intern Med J 2004;34(1–2):20–3.
11. Salive ME, Jones CA, Guralnik JM, et al. Serum creatinine levels in older adults: relationship with health status and medications. Age Ageing 1995;24(2):142–50.
12. Shen Y, Chen J, Chen X, et al. Prevalence and associated factors of sarcopenia in nursing home residents: a systematic review and meta-analysis. J Am Med Dir Assoc 2019;20(1):5–13.
13. Cockcroft DW, Gault MH. Prediction of creatinine clearance from serum creatinine. Nephron 1976;16(1):31–41.
14. Levey AS, Bosch JP, Lewis JB, et al. A more accurate method to estimate glomerular filtration rate from serum creatinine: a new prediction equation. Modification of Diet in Renal Disease Study Group. Ann Intern Med 1999;130(6):461–70.
15. Levey AS, Stevens LA, Schmid CH, et al. A new equation to estimate glomerular filtration rate. Ann Intern Med 2009;150(9):604–12.
16. Houlind MB, Petersen KK, Palm H, et al. Creatinine-based renal function estimates and dosage of postoperative pain management for elderly acute hip fracture patients. Pharmaceuticals (Basel) 2018;11(3) [pii:E88].
17. Hirst JA, Montes MDV, Taylor CJ, et al. Impact of a single eGFR and eGFR-estimating equation on chronic kidney disease reclassification: a cohort study in primary care. Br J Gen Pract 2018;68(673):e524–30.
18. Verhave JC, Fesler P, Ribstein J, et al. Estimation of renal function in subjects with normal serum creatinine levels: influence of age and body mass index. Am J Kidney Dis 2005;46(2):233–41.

19. Lamb EJ, Webb MC, Abbas NA. The significance of serum troponin T in patients with kidney disease: a review of the literature. Ann Clin Biochem 2004;41(Pt 1): 1–9.

20. Lamb EJ, Wood J, Stowe HJ, et al. Susceptibility of glomerular filtration rate estimations to variations in creatinine methodology: a study in older patients. Ann Clin Biochem 2005;42(Pt 1):11–8.

21. Romagnani P, Remuzzi G, Glassock R, et al. Chronic kidney disease. Nat Rev Dis Primers 2017;3:17088.

22. Guralnik JM, Eisenstaedt RS, Ferrucci L, et al. Prevalence of anemia in persons 65 years and older in the United States: evidence for a high rate of unexplained anemia. Blood 2004;104(8):2263–8.

23. Harman SM, Metter EJ, Tobin JD, et al, Baltimore Longitudinal Study of A. Longitudinal effects of aging on serum total and free testosterone levels in healthy men. Baltimore Longitudinal Study of Aging. J Clin Endocrinol Metab 2001;86(2): 724–31.

24. Weber JP, Walsh PC, Peters CA, et al. Effect of reversible androgen deprivation on hemoglobin and serum immunoreactive erythropoietin in men. Am J Hematol 1991;36(3):190–4.

25. Yancik R, Ershler W, Satariano W, et al. Report of the national institute on aging task force on comorbidity. J Gerontol A Biol Sci Med Sci 2007;62(3):275–80.

26. Ershler WB, Sheng S, McKelvey J, et al. Serum erythropoietin and aging: a longitudinal analysis. J Am Geriatr Soc 2005;53(8):1360–5.

27. Kario K, Matsuo T, Kodama K, et al. Reduced erythropoietin secretion in senile anemia. Am J Hematol 1992;41(4):252–7.

28. Artz AS, Fergusson D, Drinka PJ, et al. Mechanisms of unexplained anemia in the nursing home. J Am Geriatr Soc 2004;52(3):423–7.

29. Carpenter MA, Kendall RG, O'Brien AE, et al. Reduced erythropoietin response to anaemia in elderly patients with normocytic anaemia. Eur J Haematol 1992;49(3): 119–21.

30. Goodnough LT, Price TH, Parvin CA. The endogenous erythropoietin response and the erythropoietic response to blood loss anemia: the effects of age and gender. J Lab Clin Med 1995;126(1):57–64.

31. Joosten E, Van Hove L, Lesaffre E, et al. Serum erythropoietin levels in elderly inpatients with anemia of chronic disorders and iron deficiency anemia. J Am Geriatr Soc 1993;41(12):1301–4.

32. McClellan W, Aronoff SL, Bolton WK, et al. The prevalence of anemia in patients with chronic kidney disease. Curr Med Res Opin 2004;20(9):1501–10.

33. Powers JS, Krantz SB, Collins JC, et al. Erythropoietin response to anemia as a function of age. J Am Geriatr Soc 1991;39(1):30–2.

34. Zauber NP, Zauber AG. Hematologic data of healthy very old people. JAMA 1987;257(16):2181–4.

35. Ble A, Fink JC, Woodman RC, et al. Renal function, erythropoietin, and anemia of older persons: the InCHIANTI study. Arch Intern Med 2005;165(19):2222–7.

36. Greco A, Paroni G, Seripa D, et al. Frailty, disability and physical exercise in the aging process and in chronic kidney disease. Kidney Blood Press Res 2014; 39(2–3):164–8.

37. Culleton BF, Manns BJ, Zhang J, et al. Impact of anemia on hospitalization and mortality in older adults. Blood 2006;107(10):3841–6.

38. Li S, Foley RN, Collins AJ. Anemia and cardiovascular disease, hospitalization, end stage renal disease, and death in older patients with chronic kidney disease. Int Urol Nephrol 2005;37(2):395–402.

39. Kurella M, Chertow GM, Fried LF, et al. Chronic kidney disease and cognitive impairment in the elderly: the health, aging, and body composition study. J Am Soc Nephrol 2005;16(7):2127–33.
40. Lefebvre P, Duh MS, Buteau S, et al. Medical costs of untreated anemia in elderly patients with predialysis chronic kidney disease. J Am Soc Nephrol 2006;17(12):3497–502.
41. Eschbach JW, Abdulhadi MH, Browne JK, et al. Recombinant human erythropoietin in anemic patients with end-stage renal disease. Results of a phase III multicenter clinical trial. Ann Intern Med 1989;111(12):992–1000.
42. Eschbach JW, Egrie JC, Downing MR, et al. Correction of the anemia of end-stage renal disease with recombinant human erythropoietin. Results of a combined phase I and II clinical trial. N Engl J Med 1987;316(2):73–8.
43. Ling B, Walczyk M, Agarwal A, et al. Darbepoetin alfa administered once monthly maintains hemoglobin concentrations in patients with chronic kidney disease. Clin Nephrol 2005;63(5):327–34.
44. Locatelli F, Del Vecchio L, Marai P. Clinical experience with darbepoetin-alfa (Aranesp). Contrib Nephrol 2002;(137):403–7.
45. Macdougall IC. CERA (Continuous Erythropoietin Receptor Activator): a new erythropoiesis-stimulating agent for the treatment of anemia. Curr Hematol Rep 2005;4(6):436–40.
46. Macdougall IC. Recent advances in erythropoietic agents in renal anemia. Semin Nephrol 2006;26(4):313–8.
47. Rainville N, Jachimowicz E, Wojchowski DM. Targeting EPO and EPO receptor pathways in anemia and dysregulated erythropoiesis. Expert Opin Ther Targets 2016;20(3):287–301.
48. Nordstrom BL, Luo W, Fraeman K, et al. Use of erythropoiesis-stimulating agents among chemotherapy patients with hemoglobin exceeding 12 grams per deciliter. J Manag Care Pharm 2008;14(9):858–69.
49. Shank WA Jr, Balducci L. Recombinant hemopoietic growth factors: comparative hemopoietic response in younger and older subjects. J Am Geriatr Soc 1992;40(2):151–4.
50. Nicholas JC. A study of the response of elderly patients with end-stage renal disease to epoetin alfa or beta. Drugs Aging 2004;21(3):187–201.
51. Delano BG. Improvements in quality of life following treatment with r-HuEPO in anemic hemodialysis patients. Am J Kidney Dis 1989;14(2 Suppl 1):14–8.
52. Moreno F, Aracil FJ, Perez R, et al. Controlled study on the improvement of quality of life in elderly hemodialysis patients after correcting end-stage renal disease-related anemia with erythropoietin. Am J Kidney Dis 1996;27(4):548–56.
53. Besarab A, Bolton WK, Browne JK, et al. The effects of normal as compared with low hematocrit values in patients with cardiac disease who are receiving hemodialysis and epoetin. N Engl J Med 1998;339(9):584–90.
54. Singh AK, Szczech L, Tang KL, et al. Correction of anemia with epoetin alfa in chronic kidney disease. N Engl J Med 2006;355(20):2085–98.
55. Drueke TB, Locatelli F, Clyne N, et al. Normalization of hemoglobin level in patients with chronic kidney disease and anemia. N Engl J Med 2006;355(20):2071–84.
56. Levin A, Djurdjev O, Thompson C, et al. Canadian randomized trial of hemoglobin maintenance to prevent or delay left ventricular mass growth in patients with CKD. Am J Kidney Dis 2005;46(5):799–811.
57. Roger SD, McMahon LP, Clarkson A, et al. Effects of early and late intervention with epoetin alpha on left ventricular mass among patients with chronic kidney

disease (stage 3 or 4): results of a randomized clinical trial. J Am Soc Nephrol 2004;15(1):148–56.

58. KDIGO Anemia Work Group. KDIGO clinical practice guidelines for anemia in CKD. Kidney Int Suppl 2012;2(4):279–331.

59. Kliger AS, Foley RN, Goldfarb DS, et al. KDOQI US Commentary on the 2012 clinical practice guidelines for anemia in CKD. Am J Kidney Dis 2013;62(5):849–59.

60. FDA. Drug Safety Communication: modified dosing recommendations to improve the safe use of Erythropoiesis-Stimulating Agents (ESAs) in chronic kidney disease. Available at: https://www.fda.gov/Drugs/DrugSafety/ucm259639.htm. Accessed January 21, 2019.

61. Pfeffer MA, Burdmann EA, Chen CY, et al. A trial of darbepoetin alfa in type 2 diabetes and chronic kidney disease. N Engl J Med 2009;361(21):2019–32.

Inflammatory Pathways to Anemia in the Frail Elderly

Juliette Tavenier, MSc[a], Sean X. Leng, MD, PhD[b],*

KEYWORDS

- Anemia • Frailty • Inflammation • Older adults

KEY POINTS

- Anemia is a contributing factor to frailty; both are common geriatric syndromes that interact with each other, leading to adverse health outcomes and early mortality.
- Anemia and frailty share pathophysiologic mechanisms involving chronic inflammation.
- Chronic inflammation may contribute to the pathogenesis of anemia in the frail elderly through impaired iron metabolism, reduced erythropoiesis, and shortened erythrocyte lifespan.
- Understanding the role of inflammation in the development of anemia and frailty will help reveal pathways that may serve as potential targets for novel prevention and treatment strategies.

INTRODUCTION

Anemia is a common condition defined by reduced hemoglobin levels. Using the World Health Organization threshold of greater than 12 g/dL for women and greater than 13 g/dL for men, the prevalence of anemia ranges from 8.1% to 24.7% in community-dwelling older adults aged 65 years and older.[1] Anemia is a risk factor for adverse health outcomes, including frailty, falls, and early mortality.[2–4] The pathophysiologic effects of reduced hemoglobin, such as fatigue, and decreased muscle strength and physical function, which are also cardinal features of frailty, suggest a close relationship between anemia and frailty.[4–6] An important contributing factor to the pathogenesis of frailty is an age-associated state of chronic, low-grade inflammation or inflammaging.[7] A link between chronic inflammation, anemia, and frailty has previously been suggested.[8,9] The authors review the evidence for the role of chronic inflammation in anemia with a focus on their tie to frailty in older adults.

Disclosure Statement: The authors have nothing to disclose.
[a] Clinical Research Centre, Copenhagen University Hospital Hvidovre, Kettegaard Alle 30, Hvidovre 2650, Denmark; [b] Division of Geriatric Medicine and Gerontology, Department of Medicine, Johns Hopkins University School of Medicine, 5501 Hopkins Bayview Circle – Room 1A.38A, Baltimore, MD 21224, USA
* Corresponding author.
E-mail address: sleng1@jhmi.edu

FRAILTY

Frailty is a widely recognized clinical syndrome in older adults and is a risk factor for adverse health outcomes, including falls, hospitalization, disability, and early mortality.[10] Conceptually, frailty is described as a state of increased vulnerability resulting from age-related decline in the physiologic reserve and function of multiple organ systems. Several constructs have been proposed to assess frailty and have recently been reviewed.[11] The most used frailty instruments are the physical frailty phenotype developed in the Cardiovascular Health Study by Fried and colleagues[10] and the deficit accumulation index developed by Mitnitski, Mogilner, and Rockwood.[12]

The physical frailty phenotype defines frailty using the following criteria: unintentional weight loss, slowness, weakness, exhaustion, and physical inactivity.[10] Individuals with 3 or more of the criteria are classified as frail, those with 1 to 2 criteria as prefrail, and those with none of the 5 criteria as nonfrail. In contrast, the deficit accumulation index is based on the ratio of deficits (symptoms, disease, and abnormal laboratory test) to the total number of evaluated parameters. Because frailty index and its variations include many parameters of diseases and disability, they are not ideal for investigating the cause of frailty.

In the following sections, the authors focus on the physical frailty phenotype and provide an overview of current evidence suggesting inflammatory pathways to anemia and frailty in older adults.

CHRONIC INFLAMMATION

In 2000, Claudio Franceschi coined the term "inflammaging" to describe the age-related state of chronic, low-grade inflammation.[7] Since then, the role of inflammaging in the development and progression of anemia, cardiovascular disease, type 2 diabetes, neurodegenerative disease, frailty, disability, and early mortality has been actively studied.[13-15]

Assessing Chronic Inflammation

Inflammaging differs from acute inflammatory responses in that it is a low-grade, systemic, unresolved, and smoldering chronic inflammation clearly demonstrated by a 2- to 4-fold increase in serum levels of acute phase proteins and/or proinflammatory cytokines in the absence of overt infection or injury. A gold standard for the assessment or diagnosis of chronic inflammation is still lacking, and thus a wide variety of biomarkers such as cytokines and chemokines, including members of the interleukin (IL)-1 family, IL-6, IL-8, IL-18, and tumor necrosis factor (TNF)-α, are commonly used. White blood cell (WBC) counts and C-reactive protein (CRP) have also been traditionally used to assess chronic inflammation. IL-6 has received particular attention due to its strong associations with age-related conditions and mortality.[16] Several attempts have been made to optimize the assessment of chronic inflammation.[17,18] An inflammation score developed in the InCHIANTI and Cardiovascular Health Study revealed that out of 15 nuclear factor kappa B–mediated pathway markers of inflammation, IL-6 and TNF receptor I (TNF-RI) were the most informative with regard to age-related chronic inflammation and mortality risk in older adults.[17] Other potential biomarkers of chronic inflammation are emerging, such as soluble urokinase plasminogen activator receptor (suPAR). Like other commonly used inflammatory biomarkers, suPAR is elevated in a wide range of chronic conditions and is associated with disease severity and mortality.[19-21] In addition, suPAR has the advantage of being only minimally affected by acute stimuli and circadian fluctuation in contrast to cytokines and acute phase proteins and, therefore, has the potential for use as a more reliable biomarker of chronic inflammation.[22,23] suPAR levels are correlated with WBC counts and levels of CRP and IL-6.[24]

Chronic Inflammation and Frailty

Cross-sectional data from large cohort studies of older adults demonstrate that increased IL-6, CRP, TNF-α, TNF-RI, and TNF-RII levels as well as total WBC, neutrophil, and monocyte counts were directly associated with physical frailty phenotype.[13,25–28] In longitudinal studies, elevated CRP levels and WBC, neutrophil, and monocyte counts predicted incident frailty.[29,30] Moreover, elevated levels of immune activation markers such as neopterin are associated with frailty in community-dwelling older individuals, independently of IL-6 levels.[31] Monocytes of frail older adults have upregulated ex vivo expression of stress-responsive inflammatory pathway genes and upregulated expression of the proinflammatory chemokine CXCL10.[32,33] Frail older adults were also reported to have changes in the numbers and function of lymphocyte populations, including increased production of IL-6 by the peripheral blood mononuclear cells, higher frequencies of proinflammatory CCR5+ T cells, and elevated proportions of highly differentiated (CD28⁻) CD4 and CD8 T cells.[34–37] These findings suggest that immune activation may be a precipitating factor for chronic inflammation and the development of frailty.

In addition to the direct associations with frailty described earlier, chronic inflammation may be involved indirectly in the pathogenesis of frailty through deleterious effects on different physiologic systems (**Fig. 1**). In frail older adults, elevated IL-6 levels and WBC counts are inversely associated with insulin-like growth factor (IGF)-1 and hemoglobin levels, and low IGF-1 and hemoglobin levels were independently associated with frailty.[26,38] Chronic inflammation also contributes to dysregulation of the musculoskeletal system. For example, elevated levels of IL-6, CRP, TNF-α, TNF-RI, and

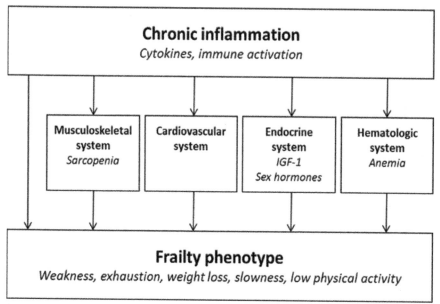

Fig. 1. Pathogenesis of the frailty syndrome: direct and indirect effects of chronic inflammation and relationship with anemia.

suPAR are associated with decreased muscle mass and strength in older persons.[39–41]

ANEMIA IN THE CONTEXT OF FRAILTY AND CHRONIC INFLAMMATION
Anemia in Frailty

Multiple studies have shown an increased prevalence of anemia in the frail elderly.[4,42] Frailty is also associated with reduced hemoglobin levels in older adults.[2,26,42,43] Moreover, low hemoglobin levels, although still within the normal range, were associated with frailty.[4] In a longitudinal study in older men, the presence of anemia preceded frailty, supporting the hypothesis that anemia is a risk factor for frailty.[44]

Anemia could contribute to frailty through a reduction in oxygen delivery to muscles impairing muscle strength and function.[45] The effects of reduced hemoglobin, such as fatigue, and decreased muscle strength and physical function are consistent with clinical features of frailty.[5,6,46] Low hemoglobin was associated with weight loss in men and with reduced grip strength and gait speed in women.[47]

The pathophysiology of anemia in the frail elderly remains unclear and studies exploring the mechanisms of anemia in frailty are scarce. However, inflammaging associated with frailty may serve as an important mechanism.[8] In older adults, low hemoglobin was found to be associated with chronic inflammation.[2,48] In particular, decreased hemoglobin was associated with elevated IL-6 levels in frail older individuals rather than in nonfrail individuals.[26] Interestingly, reduced monocyte numbers were also associated with anemia.[49] Because monocytes and erythrocyte share a common myeloid progenitor, this observation may suggest the involvement of reduced myelopoiesis in the development of anemia. Anemia of chronic inflammation accounts for one-quarter of all subtypes of anemia commonly seen in older adults. Levels of IL-6, CRP, and TNF-α are elevated in anemia of chronic inflammation.[50–52] Chronic inflammation may contribute to the pathogenesis of anemia through several mechanisms: (1) impairment of iron metabolism (upregulation of hepcidin and iron retention in macrophages, duodenal epithelial cells, and liver cells), (2) reduced erythropoiesis (inhibition of proliferation of erythroid precursor cells and/or increased erythropoietin resistance), and (3) shortened erythrocyte lifespan (**Fig. 2**).

Impairment of Iron Metabolism

Hepcidin is essential in the regulation of iron metabolism; it reduces circulating iron through degradation of ferroportin, the only known cellular iron exporter, through binding and internalization.[53] This leads to the retention of dietary iron in duodenal enterocytes, recycled iron from senescent erythrocytes in macrophages, and stored iron in hepatocytes.[54] Hepcidin gene HAMP is downregulated by erythroferrone and upregulated by iron levels and by inflammation, namely by IL-6 signaling through STAT3 pathway and activin B through SMAD signaling.[54] Hepcidin levels in older adults, particularly those who are frail, have yet to be adequately evaluated. In the Leiden 85-Plus Study, plasma hepcidin levels were elevated in participants with anemia of chronic inflammation, and elevated hepcidin levels were correlated with CRP and erythropoietin levels.[51] In contrast, in the InCHIANTI study, urinary hepcidin levels were reduced in patients with anemia of chronic inflammation and were not correlated with IL-6 and CRP levels.[52] This lack of consistency could be explained by different methods and biofluids for measurement of hepcidin if there was a role of hepcidin in the relationship between chronic inflammation and reduced iron. Another possibility

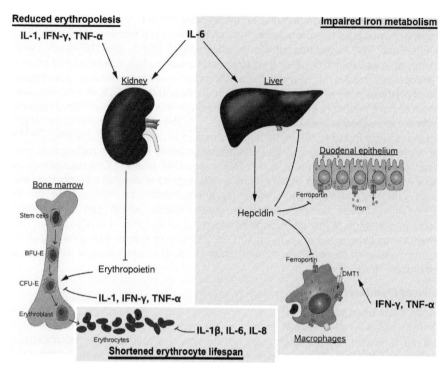

Fig. 2. Inflammatory pathways to anemia. Chronic inflammation may contribute to the development of anemia through impairment of iron metabolism by upregulation of hepcidin and divalent metal transporter 1 iron transporter, leading to iron retention in macrophages and liver stores and reduce uptake of dietary iron. It may also affect erythrocyte life cycle through reduction of erythropoiesis, erythropoietin resistance, and decreased erythrocyte survival.

could be a direct effect of chronic inflammation on ferroportin. To this end, large-scale and more in-depth studies are needed to elucidate the role of hepcidin in anemia of chronic inflammation in older adults.

Macrophage also plays an important role in iron metabolism. Macrophages phagocytose senescent erythrocytes and release iron into the plasma. This iron recycling accounts for 90% of the daily iron requirements for hemoglobin synthesis and erythropoiesis. In addition to the effect of hepcidin on ferroportin, interferon gamma (IFN-γ) and lipopolysaccharide (LPS) were found to downregulate ferroportin messenger RNA in activated macrophages, further increasing iron sequestration in macrophages.[55] Moreover, macrophages activated by IFN-γ, TNF-α, or LPS upregulate the expression of divalent metal transporter 1, a transmembrane iron transporter, leading to increased ferrous iron uptake by macrophages.[55]

The iron sequestration resulted from increased hepcidin can cause hypoferremia and iron-restricted erythropoiesis. Moreover, chronic inflammation may also have a direct effect on erythropoiesis as described next.

Reduced Erythropoiesis

The development and maturation of burst-forming unit-erythroid, colony-forming unit-erythroid, and erythroid precursor cells depends on erythropoietin signaling through erythropoietin receptor. Early studies showed that IL-1, TNF-α, and IFN-γ affect development of colony-forming unit-erythroid cells.[56,57] IFN-γ also induces erythroid progenitor apoptosis by upregulating the expression of proapoptotic molecules such as Fas–FasL, TNF-related apoptosis-inducing ligand, CD95, and TNF-related weak inducer of apoptosis.[58,59] Other mechanisms of inflammation-mediated reduction of erythropoiesis involve IFN-γ–mediated erythropoietin resistance through downregulation of erythropoietin receptors.[60] In addition, IL-1α and β, IFN-γ, IL-6, and TNF were shown to have inhibitory effects on erythropoietin production in vitro.[61] Erythropoietin levels are increased in anemia of inflammation.[51] In the InCHIANTI cohort, erythropoietin levels were found to be unaffected or elevated in anemia of inflammation.[50,52] In the same cohort, progressively low erythropoietin levels in anemic participants were associated with increasing IL-6, IL-1β, TNF-α, and CRP levels.[48] One possible explanation to these contrasting observations is that anemia of chronic inflammation may begin with high erythropoietin levels as a mechanism to compensate for the inflammation-related downregulation of erythropoiesis, which can subsequently evolve into a stage of low erythropoietin when the production of erythropoietin fails, either due to exhaustion of erythropoietin production or due to strengthening of the inhibitory effect of chronic inflammation, thus resulting in overt anemia with reduced hemoglobin levels.[48]

Reduced Erythrocyte Lifespan

Finally, it has been suggested that oxidative stress associated with chronic inflammation is involved in red blood cell shrinkage and eryptosis.[62] Incubation with low levels of IL-1β, IL-6, and IL-8 led to changes reminiscing of eryptosis in the morphology of erythrocytes and that CRP caused eryptosis.[63,64] Oxidative stress causes deformability of red blood cells, leading to increased phagocytosis by macrophages.[65] Studies in rats have shown that TNF-α and IL-1 injections reduced erythrocyte lifespan and synthesis, resulting in the development of anemia.[66] In a small study comparing elderly to young individuals, older persons had a greater prevalence of anemia and increased numbers of apoptotic erythrocytes.[67] This increased erythrocyte death may not be compensated due to the reduced erythropoiesis.

SUMMARY

Evidence suggests that chronic inflammation may be a common pathway leading to anemia and frailty in the elderly. However, the exact mechanisms remain to be elucidated. Anemia is a condition commonly seen in older adults. It has a complex pathophysiology and is intertwined with frailty. Frailty is a common geriatric syndrome. Its adverse impact on the health of older adults is well established. Further clinical studies in humans are needed to gain a better understanding of the role of chronic inflammation in contributing to anemia in the frail elderly. These studies will pave the way for the development of novel interventional strategies for the prevention and treatment of anemia and, likely, also frailty in older adults.

REFERENCES

1. Patel KV. Epidemiology of anemia in older adults. Semin Hematol 2008;45(4): 210–7.
2. Zakai NA, Katz R, Hirsch C, et al. A prospective study of anemia status, hemoglobin concentration, and mortality in an elderly cohort: the cardiovascular health study. Arch Intern Med 2005;165(19):2214–20.
3. Penninx BWJH, Pluijm SMF, Lips P, et al. Late-life anemia is associated with increased risk of recurrent falls. J Am Geriatr Soc 2005;53(12):2106–11.

4. Chaves PHM, Semba RD, Leng SX, et al. Impact of anemia and cardiovascular disease on frailty status of community-dwelling older women: the Women's Health and Aging Studies I and II. J Gerontol A Biol Sci Med Sci 2005;60(6):729–35.
5. Penninx BWJH, Pahor M, Cesari M, et al. Anemia is associated with disability and decreased physical performance and muscle strength in the elderly. J Am Geriatr Soc 2004;52(5):719–24.
6. Cesari M, Penninx BWJH, Lauretani F, et al. Hemoglobin levels and skeletal muscle: results from the InCHIANTI study. J Gerontol A Biol Sci Med Sci 2004;59(3):249–54.
7. Franceschi C, Bonafè M, Valensin S, et al. Inflamm-aging: an evolutionary perspective on immunosenescence. Ann N Y Acad Sci 2000;908:244–54.
8. Ershler WB. Biological interactions of aging and anemia: a focus on cytokines. J Am Geriatr Soc 2003;51(3 Suppl):S18–21.
9. Roy CN. Anemia in frailty. Clin Geriatr Med 2011;27(1):67–78.
10. Fried LP, Tangen CM, Walston J, et al. Frailty in older adults: evidence for a phenotype. J Gerontol A Biol Sci Med Sci 2001;56(3):M146–56.
11. Buta BJ, Walston JD, Godino JG, et al. Frailty assessment instruments: systematic characterization of the uses and contexts of highly-cited instruments. Ageing Res Rev 2016;26:53–61.
12. Mitnitski AB, Mogilner AJ, Rockwood K. Accumulation of deficits as a proxy measure of aging. ScientificWorldJournal 2001;1:323–36.
13. Leng SX, Xue Q-L, Tian J, et al. Inflammation and frailty in older women. J Am Geriatr Soc 2007;55(6):864–71.
14. Franceschi C, Campisi J. Chronic inflammation (inflammaging) and its potential contribution to age-associated diseases. J Gerontol A Biol Sci Med Sci 2014;69(Suppl 1):S4–9.
15. Michaud M, Balardy L, Moulis G, et al. Proinflammatory cytokines, aging, and age-related diseases. J Am Med Dir Assoc 2013;14(12):877–82.
16. Ershler WB, Keller ET. Age-associated increased interleukin-6 gene expression, late-life diseases, and frailty. Annu Rev Med 2000;51:245–70.
17. Varadhan R, Yao W, Matteini A, et al. Simple biologically informed inflammatory index of two serum cytokines predicts 10 Year all-cause mortality in older adults. J Gerontol A Biol Sci Med Sci 2014;69A(2):165–73.
18. Bandeen-Roche K, Walston JD, Huang Y, et al. Measuring systemic inflammatory regulation in older adults: evidence and utility. Rejuvenation Res 2009;12(6):403–10.
19. Haupt TH, Petersen J, Ellekilde G, et al. Plasma suPAR levels are associated with mortality, admission time, and Charlson Comorbidity Index in the acutely admitted medical patient: a prospective observational study. Crit Care 2012;16(4):R130.
20. Rasmussen LJH, Ladelund S, Haupt TH, et al. Soluble urokinase plasminogen activator receptor (suPAR) in acute care: a strong marker of disease presence and severity, readmission and mortality. A retrospective cohort study. Emerg Med J EMJ 2016;33(11):769–75.
21. Eugen-Olsen J, Andersen O, Linneberg A, et al. Circulating soluble urokinase plasminogen activator receptor predicts cancer, cardiovascular disease, diabetes and mortality in the general population. J Intern Med 2010;268:296–308.
22. Koch A, Voigt S, Kruschinski C, et al. Circulating soluble urokinase plasminogen activator receptor is stably elevated during the first week of treatment in the intensive care unit and predicts mortality in critically ill patients. Crit Care 2011;15(1):R63.

23. Andersen O, Eugen-Olsen J, Kofoed K, et al. Soluble urokinase plasminogen activator receptor is a marker of dysmetabolism in HIV-infected patients receiving highly active antiretroviral therapy. J Med Virol 2008;80:209–16.

24. Rasmussen LJH, Moffitt TE, Eugen-Olsen J, et al. Cumulative childhood risk is associated with a new measure of chronic inflammation in adulthood. J Child Psychol Psychiatry 2019;60(2):199–208.

25. Leng SX, Xue Q-L, Tian J, et al. Associations of neutrophil and monocyte counts with frailty in community-dwelling disabled older women: results from the Women's Health and Aging Studies I. Exp Gerontol 2009;44(8):511–6.

26. Leng S, Chaves P, Koenig K, et al. Serum interleukin-6 and hemoglobin as physiological correlates in the geriatric syndrome of frailty: a pilot study. J Am Geriatr Soc 2002;50(7):1268–71.

27. Walston J, McBurnie MA, Newman A, et al. Frailty and activation of the inflammation and coagulation systems with and without clinical comorbidities: results from the Cardiovascular Health Study. Arch Intern Med 2002;162(20):2333–41.

28. Valdiglesias V, Marcos-Pérez D, Lorenzi M, et al. Immunological alterations in frail older adults: a cross sectional study. Exp Gerontol 2018;112:119–26.

29. Walker KA, Walston J, Gottesman RF, et al. Midlife systemic inflammation is associated with frailty in later life: the ARIC study. J Gerontol A Biol Sci Med Sci 2019; 74(3):343–9.

30. Gale CR, Baylis D, Cooper C, et al. Inflammatory markers and incident frailty in men and women: the English Longitudinal Study of Ageing. Age (Dordr) 2013; 35(6):2493–501.

31. Leng SX, Tian X, Matteini A, et al. IL-6-independent association of elevated serum neopterin levels with prevalent frailty in community-dwelling older adults. Age Ageing 2011;40(4):475–81.

32. Qu T, Walston JD, Yang H, et al. Upregulated ex vivo expression of stress-responsive inflammatory pathway genes by LPS-challenged CD14(+) monocytes in frail older adults. Mech Ageing Dev 2009;130(3):161–6.

33. Qu T, Yang H, Walston JD, et al. Upregulated monocytic expression of CXC chemokine ligand 10 (CXCL-10) and its relationship with serum interleukin-6 levels in the syndrome of frailty. Cytokine 2009;46(3):319–24.

34. Leng SX, Yang H, Walston JD. Decreased cell proliferation and altered cytokine production in frail older adults. Aging Clin Exp Res 2004;16(3):249–52.

35. De Fanis U, Wang GC, Fedarko NS, et al. T-lymphocytes expressing CC chemokine receptor-5 are increased in frail older adults. J Am Geriatr Soc 2008;56(5): 904–8.

36. Semba RD, Margolick JB, Leng S, et al. T cell subsets and mortality in older community-dwelling women. Exp Gerontol 2005;40:81–7.

37. Ng TP, Camous X, Nyunt MSZ, et al. Markers of T-cell senescence and physical frailty: insights from Singapore Longitudinal Ageing Studies. NPJ Aging Mech Dis 2015;1:15005.

38. Leng SX, Hung W, Cappola AR, et al. White blood cell counts, insulin-like growth factor-1 levels, and frailty in community-dwelling older women. J Gerontol A Biol Sci Med Sci 2009;64(4):499–502.

39. Visser M, Pahor M, Taaffe DR, et al. Relationship of interleukin-6 and tumor necrosis factor-alpha with muscle mass and muscle strength in elderly men and women: the Health ABC Study. J Gerontol A Biol Sci Med Sci 2002;57:M326–32.

40. Schaap LA, Pluijm SMF, Deeg DJH, et al. Higher inflammatory marker levels in older persons: associations with 5-year change in muscle mass and muscle strength. J Gerontol A Biol Sci Med Sci 2009;64A(11):1183–9.

41. Klausen HH, Bodilsen AC, Petersen J, et al. How inflammation underlies physical and organ function in acutely admitted older medical patients. Mech Ageing Dev 2017;164:67–75.

42. Fried LP, Xue Q-L, Cappola AR, et al. Nonlinear multisystem physiological dysregulation associated with frailty in older women: implications for etiology and treatment. J Gerontol A Biol Sci Med Sci 2009;64(10):1049–57.

43. Hubbard RE, Sinead O'Mahony M, Woodhouse KW. Erythropoietin and anemia in aging and frailty. J Am Geriatr Soc 2008;56(11):2164–5.

44. Hirani V, Naganathan V, Blyth F, et al. Cross-sectional and longitudinal associations between anemia and frailty in older Australian men: the concord health and aging in men project. J Am Med Dir Assoc 2015;16(7):614–20.

45. Ng TP, Lu Y, Choo RWM, et al. Dysregulated homeostatic pathways in sarcopenia among frail older adults. Aging Cell 2018;17:e12842.

46. Chaves PHM, Ashar B, Guralnik JM, et al. Looking at the relationship between hemoglobin concentration and prevalent mobility difficulty in older women. Should the criteria currently used to define anemia in older people be reevaluated? J Am Geriatr Soc 2002;50(7):1257–64.

47. Silva JC, Moraes ZV, Silva C, et al. Understanding red blood cell parameters in the context of the frailty phenotype: interpretations of the FIBRA (Frailty in Brazilian Seniors) study. Arch Gerontol Geriatr 2014;59(3):636–41.

48. Ferrucci L, Guralnik JM, Woodman RC, et al. Proinflammatory state and circulating erythropoietin in persons with and without anemia. Am J Med 2005;118(11):1288.

49. Verschoor CP, Johnstone J, Millar J, et al. Alterations to the frequency and function of peripheral blood monocytes and associations with chronic disease in the advanced-age, frail elderly. PLoS One 2014;9(8):e104522.

50. Ferrucci L, Guralnik JM, Bandinelli S, et al. Unexplained anaemia in older persons is characterised by low erythropoietin and low levels of pro-inflammatory markers. Br J Haematol 2007;136(6):849–55.

51. den Elzen WPJ, de Craen AJM, Wiegerinck ET, et al. Plasma hepcidin levels and anemia in old age. The Leiden 85-Plus Study. Haematologica 2013;98(3):448–54.

52. Ferrucci L, Semba RD, Guralnik JM, et al. Proinflammatory state, hepcidin, and anemia in older persons. Blood 2010;115(18):3810–6.

53. Nemeth E, Tuttle MS, Powelson J, et al. Hepcidin regulates cellular iron efflux by binding to ferroportin and inducing its internalization. Science 2004;306(5704):2090–3.

54. Ganz T, Nemeth E. Iron homeostasis in host defence and inflammation. Nat Rev Immunol 2015;15(8):500–10.

55. Ludwiczek S, Aigner E, Theurl I, et al. Cytokine-mediated regulation of iron transport in human monocytic cells. Blood 2003;101(10):4148–54.

56. Rusten LS, Jacobsen SE. Tumor necrosis factor (TNF)-alpha directly inhibits human erythropoiesis in vitro: role of p55 and p75 TNF receptors. Blood 1995;85(4):989–96.

57. Means RT, Dessypris EN, Krantz SB. Inhibition of human erythroid colony-forming units by interleukin-1 is mediated by gamma interferon. J Cell Physiol 1992;150(1):59–64.

58. Dai C-H, Price JO, Brunner T, et al. Fas ligand is present in human erythroid colony-forming cells and interacts with Fas induced by interferon γ to produce erythroid cell apoptosis. Blood 1998;91(4):1235–42.

59. Felli N, Pedini F, Zeuner A, et al. Multiple members of the TNF superfamily contribute to IFN-γ-Mediated inhibition of erythropoiesis. J Immunol 2005; 175(3):1464–72.
60. Taniguchi S, Dai CH, Price JO, et al. Interferon gamma downregulates stem cell factor and erythropoietin receptors but not insulin-like growth factor-I receptors in human erythroid colony-forming cells. Blood 1997;90(6):2244–52.
61. Jelkmann WE, Fandrey J, Frede S, et al. Inhibition of erythropoietin production by cytokines. Implications for the anemia involved in inflammatory states. Ann N Y Acad Sci 1994;718:300–9 [discussion: 309–11].
62. Pretorius E. Erythrocyte deformability and eryptosis during inflammation, and impaired blood rheology. Clin Hemorheol Microcirc 2018;69(4):545–50.
63. Bester J, Pretorius E. Effects of IL-1β, IL-6 and IL-8 on erythrocytes, platelets and clot viscoelasticity. Sci Rep 2016;6:32188.
64. Abed M, Thiel C, Towhid ST, et al. Stimulation of erythrocyte cell membrane scrambling by C-reactive protein. Cell Physiol Biochem 2017;41(2):806–18.
65. Mohanty JG, Nagababu E, Rifkind JM. Red blood cell oxidative stress impairs oxygen delivery and induces red blood cell aging. Front Physiol 2014;5:84.
66. Moldawer LL, Marano MA, Wei H, et al. Cachectin/tumor necrosis factor-alpha alters red blood cell kinetics and induces anemia in vivo. FASEB J 1989;3(5): 1637–43.
67. Lupescu A, Bissinger R, Goebel T, et al. Enhanced suicidal erythrocyte death contributing to anemia in the elderly. Cell Physiol Biochem 2015;36(2):773–83.

A Growing Population of Older Adults with Sickle Cell Disease

Arun S. Shet, MD, PhD, Swee Lay Thein, MBBS, DSc*

KEYWORDS

- Sickle cell disease • Aging- and disease-related morbidities
- Disease-modifying therapies • Curative therapies

KEY POINTS

- Survival of patients with sickle cell disease (SCD) in well-resourced countries has improved greatly in the last 60 years; a newborn in the United States and United Kingdom can now expect to live to adulthood.
- Although survival has improved, life expectancy of SCD patients is still 20 to 30 years less than that of the general population.
- In well-resourced countries, the burden of disease has now shifted to adults, in which SCD has evolved into a debilitating disorder with complications associated with long-term chronic illness, in addition to those due to aging.
- The lag in providing resources and adequately equipping health care professionals with appropriate skills poses multiple challenges for effective management of this growing population of older adults with SCD.
- Patient outcomes are optimal when managed by a core of multidisciplinary specialists.

INTRODUCTION

Sickle cell disease (SCD) is caused by the presence of hemoglobin S (HbS, $\alpha_2\beta_2^S$). The syndrome comprises different genotypes that include homozygous S (HbSS): compound heterozygous forms of HbS with HbC (HbSC) and β-thalassemia (HbSβ^0 thalassemia and HbSβ$^+$ thalassemia). In patients of African ancestry, HbSS is the most common genotype at 65% to 70%, followed by HbSC (about 30%) and, the rest, HbSβ thalassemia.[1,2] SCD is the most common inherited blood disorder in the United States, and a major public health problem in Africa and Asia. In the United States, it affects an estimated 100,000 Americans (the vast majority are African Americans

Disclosure Statement: This research was funded by Intra-mural grant support.
Sickle Cell Branch, National Heart Lung and Blood Institute, National Institutes of Health, Building 10-CRC, 10 Center Drive, Bethesda, MD 20892, USA
* Corresponding author.
E-mail address: sl.thein@nih.gov

Clin Geriatr Med 35 (2019) 349–367
https://doi.org/10.1016/j.cger.2019.03.006
0749-0690/19/© 2019 Elsevier Inc. All rights reserved.

geriatric.theclinics.com

and the rest are of Hispanic descent), and about 1 in 365 African American new-borns.[3,4] In the past few decades, widespread implementation of newborn screening, prophylactic penicillin and vaccination, and increased health care access have contributed to improved childhood survival, now 96% to 98% in high-income countries.[5–7] As a consequence, in these better-resourced countries, the burden of disease has shifted to adults, where it has evolved into a chronic disorder with multiorgan damage and substantial morbidity. Overall, life expectancy of patients with SCD is still reduced by more than 2 decades compared with the general population, but more adults are living longer. Recent studies have estimated the median survival for patients with HbSS and Sβ⁰ thalassemia (the most severe sickle genotypes) at 58 years in the United States,[8] and 67 years in a single center in the United Kingdom.[9]

Older adults with SCD require greater support to address the many emerging disease complications as they age, in addition to the conditions related to physiologic aging.[10] The lag in recognition of this growing adult population with SCD and resultant inadequate resource allocation pose multiple challenges for managing the older patient. A further challenge is the inequity of treatment not only between high- and low-income countries but also within well-resourced countries; in the United States, most adults with SCD fail to receive recommended treatment, whereas patients in low-income countries lack access to comprehensive care considered standard in high-income countries.[11]

All patients with SCD, however mild their symptoms appear to be, are continuously undergoing some degree of chronic end-organ deterioration, the rate of development of chronic disease complications being modulated by their SCD genotype (patients with HbSC and HbS/mild beta-thalassemia exhibit less deterioration than HbSS and HbS/severe beta-thalassemia), genetic background, lifestyle, health care access, and environment. Within the genotype of HbSS, observational cohorts suggested that several factors modulate the rate of development of chronic disease complications. For instance, the largest series of 102 adults older than 60 in Jamaica identified 40 adults aged 60 to 87 years of age that were still alive. Higher fetal hemoglobin level (HbF) was associated with greater survival, and although these patients experienced fewer acute painful crises, nevertheless, their anemia and renal function progressively worsened as they aged.[12] Another insidious complication is silent ischemic cerebral infarcts that worsen cognitive function and contribute to morbidity in the older adult. A conglomerate of biomarkers or genetic markers[13,14] has been put forward to predict disease severity and mortality. However, for the individual patient, healthy lifestyle (lack of/minimal alcohol and tobacco exposure), normal body mass index, high levels of adherence to medication, and family support remain the most important determinants of longevity.[15]

Based on current survival estimates and the observation that by this age cumulative organ damage has an impact on morbidity and mortality,[16,17] the "older adult" is defined here as ≥40 years of age. Although sickle-related complications become more prevalent with aging, non-sickle-related causes should always be considered and appropriately treated, because these comorbidities interact and add to disease burden. Presented are 3 clinical vignettes to highlight important clinical issues frequently encountered when managing the older patient with SCD.

Case 1: Sickle Cell Anemia Patient on Exchange Transfusion with Iron Overload

T.W. is a 50-year-old woman with sickle cell anemia, history of ischemic stroke, severe carotid stenosis, atrial fibrillation, pulmonary embolism/deep vein thrombosis (DVT), chronic pain, chronic leg ulcers with osteomyelitis, and hepatic cirrhosis on liver biopsy. As active therapy for SCD, she is on a simple transfusion regimen to maintain her HbS less than 50% and also receives hydroxyurea (HU) combined with erythropoi-etin, but she has not been very adherent with her iron chelation therapy. On MRI screening for iron overload, she was found to have a T2* value indicating cardiac side-rosis and severe hepatic iron (a liver biopsy revealed cirrhosis with increased iron). She was admitted to the hospital for aggressive intravenous iron chelation with intravenous desferal. The patient is currently under evaluation for haploidentical stem cell transplantation.

Case 2: Sickle Cell Anemia Patient with Multiple Red Cell Alloantibodies

V.A. is a 64-year-old woman with HbSS disease on active therapy with HU and eryth-ropoietin with a history of multiple episodes of acute chest syndrome (ACS; the most recent in 2014), systemic hypertension on lisinopril, and chronic lower back pain for which she is on a stable dose of long-acting opioids. Her hemoglobin ranges from 7 to 8 g/dL; a simple transfusion regimen had been proposed, but she is noted to have developed multiple clinically significant red cell alloantibodies. In addition, she has developed transfusional hemosiderosis and is currently on deferasirox at a stable dose of 34 mg/kg/d.

Case 3: Hemoglobin SC Patient with Newly Detected Lung Infiltrate

F.E. is a 63-year-old man with hemoglobin SC disease, systemic hypertension, osteo-necrosis of the hip, chronic obstructive pulmonary disease secondary to cigarette smoke exposure, bilateral pulmonary embolism with likely chronic thromboembolic pulmonary hypertension (PH), intermittent atrial fibrillation, stroke in 2007, and pria-pism with residual impotence. In March 2018, he was diagnosed with a new lung mass and para-aortic lymphadenopathy. Just 6 months before, he had a pneumo-thorax due to spontaneous rupture of bullous emphysema. During workup for his lung mass, the patient was noted to have new onset thrombocytopenia, and over the next few months of being diagnosed with lung cancer, had an anterolateral wall myocardial infarction and died.

The 3 clinical vignettes illustrate the diverse clinical complications and issues rele-vant to medical practitioners dealing with the older adult with SCD.

PATHOPHYSIOLOGY AND SPECIFIC MORBIDITIES OF SICKLE CELL DISEASE

The central mechanism underlying the pathophysiology of SCD is polymerization of deoxy-HbS and the formation of irreversibly sickled red blood cells that trigger a cascade of events ultimately leading to acute painful vaso-occlusive episodes that are the hallmark of SCD. All patients with SCD are chronically anemic, because of ongoing hemolysis from the shortened lifespan of sickled erythrocytes (16–20 days compared with a normal lifespan of 120 days). Subsequent reperfusion of the ischemic tissue after vaso-occlusion generates free radicals and reactive oxygen species, which scavenge nitric oxide (NO). Continuing release of cell-free hemoglobin and sub-sequently heme add to depletion of NO. Chronic NO deficiency leads to platelet acti-vation, increased vascular resistance, and endothelial dysfunction contributing to the development of vasculopathy. The ongoing vasculopathy and inflammation inflict damage on various organs and impacts the patients as they live into their fourth, fifth, and even sixth decade, transforming SCD into a chronic multiorgan disorder. One of the largest and longest longitudinal studies of adult SCD showed that approximately one-half of surviving patients by their fifth decade had some form of irreversible dam-age of lungs, kidneys, brain, retina, or bones significantly affecting their quality of life.[16] **Table 1** lists the commonly recognized complications associated with SCD seen in

Table 1
Commonly recognized sickle-related complications

Complication	Definition	Comments
Pain	Acute pain, most commonly in the long bones, chest, back Chronic pain is pain lasting for >3 mo	Acute episodic pain occurs throughout life. Adults with SCD experience pain on >54% of days[100] Chronic pain occurs in >50% and about 40% of adults with SCD take daily opioids[101]
Anemia	Acute anemia: A decline in hemoglobin of 2 g/dL or more from steady-state values Chronic anemia: severity increases with age and major contributor to insidious organ dysfunction	Variety of causes, including infection (transient red cell aplasia most commonly caused by acute parvo virus B 19); acute hemolysis accompanying severe VOC, delayed transfusion reaction Other common causes of anemia to consider in older patients: iron deficiency, B12 deficiency, hypothyroidism, and anemia of inflammation
ACS	Acute onset of respiratory symptoms with features similar to pneumonia	Although less frequent, outcome is more severe in adults[30]
PH	Mean pulmonary artery pressure of >25 mm Hg at rest, measured by right heart catheterization	6.0%–10.4% prevalence during adulthood[35–37,102,103]
Heart failure	Most commonly left ventricular failure	Universal to some degree in adults older than age 30[39]
Chronic sickle lung disease	Progressive restrictive lung function deficit with fibrotic changes on high-resolution computed tomographic (CT) scan	Restrictive lung defects seen in >70% adults[104]
VTE	DVT detected by duplex ultrasonography, ventilation perfusion scintigraphy, or CT pulmonary angiography	11.2%–13.1% cumulative incidence rate in adulthood. High recurrence rates ~ 30%–40%. Contribution toward chronic thromboembolic PH. Consider indefinite anticoagulation.[40,41] Routine VTE prophylaxis during hospitalization and periods of increased thrombosis risk
Stroke	Acute cerebrovascular accident	Acute ischemic and hemorrhagic stroke. Hemorrhagic stroke affects both children and adults, 3-fold more in adults.[105] Exclude traditional risk factors for ischemic stroke: hypertension, diabetes mellitus, hyperlipidemia, atrial fibrillation and renal disease[106]

SCI	Clinically silent lesions of 3 mm or more on MRI scanning	Important contributing factor to neurocognitive deficits; 53% in adults[58]
Acute renal injury	Acute deterioration in renal function	Triggers include pain crisis, during ACS, acute drop in hemoglobin as in transient red cell aplasia. Often occurs as part of multiorgan failure
Renal failure	Deteriorating renal function, reduced concentrating ability, proteinuria, and progressive renal failure	Advanced disease (stage III–IV) in 4%–18% of adults[48]
Priapism	Unwanted painful and sustained erection of the penis for more than 4 h, often recurrent or persistent	20%–89% lifetime prevalence in boys and men[107]
AVN of bones	AVN of any bone, most commonly the femoral head and shoulder joint	>20% lifetime prevalence of symptomatic disease. Increased prevalence of asymptomatic disease[108]
Leg ulceration	Most commonly around the malleolar regions	>14% lifetime prevalence[109,110]
Cholelithiasis	Gallstones and gallbladder disease	Important genetic modifier is polymorphic (AT) repeats in promoter of UGT1A1 gene.[111] Gall bladder disease in 28% at median age of 28 y[16]
Retinopathy	Grade 1–IV retinopathy	>30% of patients.[112] Prevalence higher in HbSC[113]

both children and adults, although severity and clinical course may differ depending on patient's age. One should always consider that the older adult with SCD could also have unrelated comorbidities prevalent in the general population, that is, diabetes, systemic hypertension, and connective tissue disease, that further compound or accelerate sickle-related complications.

Pain is the most common symptom for which patients seek medical attention and the most frequent complaint of the older adults with SCD (all 3 cases experience chronic pain and receive long-term pain medication). Acute painful sickle cell crisis that results from vaso-occlusion affecting bones and joints is the commonest cause of an emergency room visit and hospitalization.[18,19] There are considerable differences in the frequency and intensity of sickle cell crises between adults and children; the average length of stay in adults was approximately 7.5 days[18] compared with 4.4 days in children.[20] In addition to vaso-occlusive crisis, osteomyelitis and septic arthritis can also give rise to acute skeletal pain, and clinical manifestations can be somewhat similar to acute painful crises. Older adults are more likely to have chronic pain, which is usually multifactorial from inflammation, central and peripheral neural sensitization, and avascular necrosis (AVN) of bone.[21] A review on multiple dimensions of chronic pain in adults with SCD reported that chronic pain occurs in at least 29% of adults, most frequently in those 25 to 44 years of age.[22] A recent study of chronic pain in twins showed that environmental factors are paramount in maintaining chronic pain.[23] The complexity of chronic pain in adults is further illustrated by the persistence of pain despite successful reversal of sickle hematology post–stem cell transplant in a subgroup that had chronic pain pretransplant.[24] Chronic pain negatively impacts quality of life, and its management can be challenging, because a significant knowledge gap exists in understanding the natural history and management of chronic pain in older adults.

Ongoing vasculopathy leads to chronic bone problems, such as osteopenia/osteoporosis, chronic arthritis, and osteonecrosis/AVN of bone.[25] The incidence of AVN in SCD could vary from 3% to 50% and is highest among patients older than 45 years of age (34.9%).[26] AVN most commonly affects the femoral head followed by the humeral head. Management of AVN is challenging given the limited evidence for standardized guidelines in most surgical procedures in SCD. Treatment options vary from conservative (eg, pain management, physical therapy, and decreased weight-bearing) to surgical (core decompression or arthroplasty). Early detection and intervention may delay progressive joint disease and improve quality of life. Total hip arthroplasty (THA) is usually reserved for patients with advanced AVN of the femur given its failure rate, although in recent years use of cementless prosthesis and joint management by an experienced surgeon and hematologist have improved outcomes of THA in SCD, prompting earlier intervention.[27,28]

Pulmonary complications account for significant morbidity and mortality in patients with SCD. Acute pulmonary complications include pneumonia, pulmonary embolism, and ACS. Although the incidence of ACS is lower in older adults compared with children (8.8 events per 100 patient-years in older adults vs 24.5 events per 100 patient-years in young children),[29,30] the severity and mortality are higher in older adults, largely because of a higher incidence of bone marrow and fat emboli in adults[31,32] and the presence of other organ comorbidities. Chronic pulmonary complications and sickle cell chronic lung disease are more prevalent in older adults and are characterized by impaired exercise tolerance, progressive heart failure, and impaired pulmonary function; causes include PH, pulmonary fibrosis, restrictive airway disease, and sleep-disordered breathing (nocturnal hypoxemia and obstructive sleep apnea).[33,34] PH, defined as mean pulmonary artery pressure ≥25 mm Hg at rest diagnosed by right heart catheterization, affects 6% to 11% of SCD adults[35–37] and is a leading cause of morbidity and early mortality.[38] Transthoracic echocardiography (ECHO) has been used as a noninvasive tool for screening for PH. Elevated cardiac output and left ventricular volume overload secondary to chronic anemia are other factors underlying the cardiopulmonary complications in patients with SCD.[39] As in other organ complications, deterioration in pulmonary function should prompt an appropriate screen for other causes, such as cancers, particularly in patients with a history of tobacco exposure (see case 3).

Venous thromboembolism (VTE) occurs in both young and older SCD patients but at a higher prevalence in the latter and is likely to have a greater effect on morbidity and mortality in the older patient.[40,41] The inherent hypercoagulability associated with SCD and other iatrogenic factors, such as placement of long-term indwelling catheters, recurrent hospitalization, hypoxia, inadequate VTE prophylaxis, and increasing age, influences thrombotic risk.[42] Although the exact mechanisms responsible for the hypercoagulable state in SCD are unclear, they appear to be directly related to abnormal expression of procoagulant, for example, tissue factor, and proadhesive molecules, for example, P-selectin. Tissue factor expression on pulmonary endothelial cells could trigger coagulation in vivo and possibly contribute to the in situ pulmonary thrombosis observed in at least 20% of individuals with ACS.[43] In addition to worsening acute sickle-related complications, thrombosis in the deep veins and pulmonary emboli contributes to chronic leg ulceration and thromboembolic PH, respectively (seen in case 3), adding to morbidity. The management of DVT and PE in SCD is similar to that of the general population and has been addressed in previous issues of the *Clinics in Geriatric Medicine* and more recently in clinical guidelines from the American Society of Hematology.[44] For unprovoked VTE in SCD patient, the optimal duration of anticoagulation remains undefined with proponents for extension beyond the traditional 3-month treatment period based on higher incidence of recurrent VTEs in this population group (a management strategy used in both cases 1 and 3). Extended duration anticoagulation is likely to be associated with a higher bleeding risk in older SCD patients and especially those exposed to concomitant antiplatelet therapy. A deeper understanding of SCD associated thrombophilia and the efficacy and risk of anticoagulant agents promise to provide considerable benefit to the population of older adults. Until such time, the benefit of long-term/indefinite anticoagulation should be reevaluated frequently in these patients.

All patients with SCD suffer some degree of renal impairment (also referred to as sickle cell nephropathy, SCN), most commonly manifested as hyperfiltration, hyposthenuria (diminished concentrating ability), and albuminuria. Microalbuminuria (defined as a urinary albumin/creatinine ratio >4.5 mg/mmol) is an early manifestation of SCN, reaching a prevalence of greater than 50% in older patients.[45] In a small number of patients (4%–12%), renal function progressively declines, leading to end-stage renal disease (ESRD) requiring renal replacement therapy.[46] Approximately one-quarter of patients older than 60 years of age have stage III–IV kidney disease, and ESRD was identified as the cause of death in 45% of patients aged 60 years or older.[47] It is important to note that no pathognomonic lesion defines SCN, and that other causes of renal disease, such as lupus nephritis and diabetic, hypertensive, hepatitis C virus or human immunodeficiency virus-associated nephropathy, should be considered in the differential.[48] Acceleration of renal impairment should prompt investigation of common comorbidities, in particular, hypertension and diabetes.[17] Observational data have shown that proteinuria responds to treatment with angiotensin-converting enzyme inhibitors or angiotensin receptor blockers, and treatment with these agents should be considered when the urine protein/creatinine ratio is persistently elevated greater than 50 mg/mmol.[49,50] Disease-modifying therapy (HU) should be considered alongside this specific treatment.[48,51] ESRD eventually requires standard renal replacement therapy, including erythropoietin-stimulating agents (ESA), dialysis, or renal transplant. The use of ESA when combined with HU, as in case 2, can be effective in controlling anemia.[48,52]

The spectrum of hepatic dysfunction (sickle hepatopathy) ranges from mildly abnormal liver function tests, self-limited cholestasis, to severe forms of sickle cell intrahepatic cholestasis and cirrhosis.[53] The overall prevalence of liver dysfunction in patients with SCD has not been well established and probably underappreciated because of the inability to discriminate abnormal liver enzymes resulting from hemolysis from those due to intrinsic liver disease. Thus, evaluating and treating any underlying and coexisting condition that can contribute to liver dysfunction is important. With the increasing use of blood transfusion, transfusional hemosiderosis is an emerging cause of liver disease (as observed in cases 1 and 2).[54]

Stroke, seizure, and transient ischemic attacks have been reported in more than 30% of SCD adults with SCD, and a history of these events correlates with early mortality.[8] Ischemic or thrombotic stroke peaks over the age of 29 years, and hemorrhagic stroke is most frequent in the 20- to 29-year-old age group.[55] Silent cerebral infarction (SCI) and incidental aneurysms are common in adults with SCD; the latter varies from 9% to 15% and tends to be multiple.[56–58] Neurocognitive impairment increases with age and can be compounded by sickle-related pathologic condition, such as SCI, moya moya, overt clinical stroke, anemia, and nocturnal hypoxia, throughout the patient's lifespan (see case 1, where deteriorating neurocognitive function could impact the informed consent process for experimental curative therapies). Non-sickle-related factors, hypertension, hyperlipidemia, cardiac disease, are likely to predispose the patient to vascular dementia, adding to the accelerative cognitive decline in older adults.[59]

MANAGEMENT
General Principles

Although therapeutic advances have altered patient morbidity and mortality, treatment-related (eg, secondary iron overload from blood transfusions) and physiologic aging-related complications present additional management challenges. Due consideration should be given in management of complications of pain and other acute clinical events (eg, stroke) when certain medications may require appropriate dose adjustments.[10] In addition, data and evidence-based guidelines are lacking for most complications.[60–62] Although treatment of the specific complications may be limited, it is prudent to optimize disease-modifying therapy (including HU or transfusion) in addition to general medical support (treatment of heart failure, correction of hypoxemia with oxygen therapy, and anticoagulation for those with thromboembolism).

When patients have a long period of stability and present with worsening of their sickle phenotype, the clinician should always be aware of new comorbidities as an explanation.[17] Coexistence of other chronic diseases, especially if poorly controlled, may lead to worsening of SCD. Similarly, the higher risk of colorectal cancer among African American individuals should prompt appropriate screening, perhaps earlier than the recommended age of 50 years. Hence, a management strategy of regular comprehensive review for early recognition, prevention, and treatment of organ damage should be an essential part of routine health care in older adults with SCD (**Box 1**). The authors recommend a multidisciplinary approach by a team of relevant specialists with supportive input from allied health professionals, including psychology and physiotherapy and referral to specialized centers if needed.

Box 1
An outline of management strategies in the older adult with sickle cell disease

I. Identify a primary care physician to coordinate total patient care

II. Comprehensive multisystem review to evaluate complications
- Pain: days off work due to pain
  i. Acute pain: Hospital admissions, frequency of pain at home
  ii. Chronic pain: Including use of opiate analgesia
- Detailed medical history/details of comorbidities
  i. Sickle related:
    1. Renal dysfunction (proteinuria, hematuria)
    2. Cardiorespiratory symptoms
    3. Cerebrovascular: Any memory concerns
    4. Leg ulcers
    5. Visual
    6. History of thrombosis and anticoagulant therapy
  ii. Nonsickle related: Diabetes, hypertension, gout
- Medication and vaccinations
- Transfusion history (to include frequency, transfusion reaction)
- Vitals (blood pressure, pulse oximetry, weight)
- Baseline laboratory testing (full blood count, biochemistry, hemolysis panel, liver panel, urinalysis)
- Investigation: ECHO, pulmonary function, sleep study

III. Evaluate for evidence of organ dysfunction
- Proteinuria ± hematuria → joint renal clinic
- ECHO, tricuspid regurgitant jet velocity ≥2.5 → joint cardiopulmonary clinic
- Liver function, evidence of intrahepatic cholestasis, → joint hepatology clinic
- Avascular necrosis → joint orthopedic clinic
- Headaches, cognitive decline → joint neurology clinic/neuropsychology assessment
- Visual symptoms → yearly ophthalmology review
- Daytime or nocturnal hypoxia → joint sleep/respiratory clinic

IV. Management of other comorbidities

V. Investigate/monitor therapy: HU, and similar

The 2 most widely available therapies for patients with SCD are HU and blood transfusion.

Disease-Modifying Therapies

Hydroxyurea

The main benefits of HU therapy are thought to accrue from induction of HbF that has an inhibitory effect on the rate of HbS polymerization. The efficacy of HU is also thought to arise from other effects, for example, reducing inflammation, suppressing leukocytosis and thrombocytosis, diminishing reactive oxygen species, and possibly by serving as an NO donor. HU is a disease-modifying treatment that reduced acute SCD complications in a placebo controlled randomized trial[63] and whose long-term use in nonrandomized studies demonstrated enhanced survival in patients with HbSS disease.[64,65] Because HU has a long-term safety profile with minimal side effects, the authors would argue that SCD patients should be offered the option of early rather than late HU treatment. HU has also recently been found to be relatively safe in settings with high infectious disease burden, increasing confidence in broadening the clinical use of this drug.[66,67]

It is therefore rather surprising that despite its clear benefits, HU therapy remains underutilized, probably because of a reluctance on the part of both patients and clinicians. Moreover, even when HU is prescribed, adherence can be below par, suggesting an important role for adherence counseling by the physician, which is often neglected. These considerations are compounded in the older adult with SCD with cognitive impairment. HU therapy in the older patient deserves a special mention: the older patient is likely to be more sensitive to HU dosage and easily susceptible to developing neutropenia, thrombocytopenia, and reticulocytopenia. HU treatment thus requires careful and more frequent monitoring in older adults compared with younger patients. The reasons for the relative sensitivity to HU myelotoxicity are not well known, but suggestions include repeated bone marrow infarcts and reduced hemopoietic reserve. In the older adult, the authors routinely initiate HU at 7.5 mg/kg/d and gently escalate the dose while carefully monitoring the absolute neutrophil, reticulocyte, and the platelet counts until reaching a maximum tolerated dose. Neutropenia (<1500/μL) and reticulocytopenia (<90,000/μL) would trigger withholding the drug and reinitiation at a lower dose. Combining HU with erythropoietin allows more aggressive HU dosing, which is required in high-risk disease and renal insufficiency both frequently encountered in the older adult with SCD (see case 1). In extreme cases, even a minimal dose of 5 mg/kg/d is not tolerated, requiring a search for alternative therapies.

Transfusion

Red blood cell transfusion of is one of the most effective therapies for patients with SCD. The rationale of blood transfusion in SCD is to (a) Improve oxygen carrying capacity of blood to tissues, and (b) Dilute concentration of circulating sickled erythrocytes to improve microvascular circulation.[68,69] Blood transfusion can be given as simple (or top-up) or as an exchange transfusion, either manually or automated using an apheresis machine. Intermittent blood transfusion may be used for treatment of acute complications or preparation of surgery, or long term to reduce the incidence and severity of sickle-related organ damage.

Randomized trials have demonstrated the efficacy of blood transfusion for primary and secondary prevention of stroke in children with SCD. Although stroke pathophysiology is likely to be different among adults and children, it seems reasonable to extrapolate these findings at least to ischemic stroke in adults. Many adults with a history of stroke in childhood or adulthood remain on exchange transfusion as secondary prevention albeit with a less stringent target HbS (<50% as opposed to <30%). It should be noted that although older adults with acute ischemic stroke may benefit from exchange transfusion (standard practice in children), thrombolysis may also be in order, particularly if there are traditional risk factors (eg, hypertension and hyperlipidemia); appropriate treatment and order of treatment require careful discussion with a stroke physician.

Given the clinical benefits, not surprisingly the use of blood transfusion therapy in the management of SCD is increasing. Clinical decisions to use transfusion for prevention of recurrent acute pain, priapism, leg ulcers, renal dysfunction and PH are based more on observation and clinical experience than evidence. Although very effective in preventing the several complications of SCD, transfusion therapy carries the risk of secondary iron overload, alloimmunization (both observed in these 3 cases), and transmission of blood-borne diseases, such as hepatitis C.[69,70]

Alloimmunization to RBC antigens is relatively more common in patients with SCD[71–73] and can lead to difficulties in sourcing appropriately matched blood products, delayed transfusion reactions triggering more vaso-occlusive crises, significant morbidities, and fatalities in some cases.[74–76] Alloimmunization to multiple RBC antigens often prompts the development of autoantibodies posing challenges of sourcing appropriately matched blood products; in many cases, the "least incompatible" blood is transfused under immunologic cover. As prevention, many blood transfusion centers use extended red cell phenotyping, with some having adopted molecular genotyping using microarray chips for red blood cell phenotype prediction, and some proposing genome sequencing.[77–79]

Recurrent blood transfusion, whether sporadic or long term,[80] also leads to iron overload that most commonly affects the liver; cardiac and endocrine siderosis are unusual in SCD.[81] MRI is a noninvasive method of measuring body iron load and should be used in those with a high annual blood transfusion rate and raised serum ferritin.[82] Iron chelation therapy should be considered in those with serum ferritin greater than 1000 µg/L and liver iron concentration of greater than 7 mg/g dry weight and chelation efficacy monitored with serial serum ferritin and MRI measurements.[83,84]

Newer treatments

In 2017, the Food and Drug Administration approved pharmacy grade L-glutamine (Endari)[85] for the reduction of acute complications of SCD in both adults and children. Being only the second drug approved for SCD treatment in the last 30 years, this news was met with much enthusiasm from the broader hematology community. However, the failure to include patients with mild renal impairment and one-third of the study population discontinuing the study drug raise concerns about the generalizability of these findings to older adults. Nevertheless, for older adults with normal kidney function experiencing acute crises ineffectively controlled by HU, addition of L-glutamine appears justifiable. Other agents currently in phase 3 clinical trials include Crizanlizumab (a P-selectin inhibitor),[86] small molecule anti-sickling agents, for example, GBT440 (Voxelotor),[87] and anti-inflammatory agents, for example, rivipansel.[88] These agents hold promise for patients failing to benefit from HU or those having severe symptoms despite HU therapy. Inducing HbF expression by targeting the DNA methyltransferase 1 with an oral combination of small molecules, decitabine and tetrahydrouridine, was safe and is now being evaluated for efficacy in a phase 2 study.[89,90] The development of novel agents and consideration of multimodality treatments raise several questions and possible concerns. One of these is whether combination therapy with a variety of agents targeting different pathophysiologic events will become the new standard, and will this approach have any impact on the chronic vascular pathobiology of SCD. Another concern is whether these novel therapies will be cost-effective in low- and middle-resource settings, and if their efficacy end points are cost-effective to justify their use in that particular setting.

Curative therapies

When neither HU nor regular blood transfusion is effective in limiting disease progression, other interventions should be considered even in the older adult with SCD.[10] These interventions include fully matched or haploidentical hematopoietic stem cell transplant (HSCT), gene therapy, or experimental drug treatment.[91–93]

The favorable outcome of HLA-identical sibling HSCT in children[94] prompts allogeneic transplantation sooner rather than later in young patients with symptomatic SCD.[95] However, outcomes are poorer in those older than 16 years,[94] using standard myeloablative conditioning. Reduction of the intensity of conditioning (nonmyeloablative) has expanded allogeneic transplantation as a treatment option for adult patients with preexisting organ dysfunction.[96] The HLA-matched sibling donors can be HbAS or HbAA, successful transplantation results in mixed chimerism with remarkably little graft-versus-host disease, and reversal of sickle hematology. The nonmyeloablative conditioning regimen developed at the authors' institution has now been adopted by several institutions.[91] However, although successful HSCT leads to resolution of pain in most adult SCD patients, those with chronic pain and no identifiable contributory sickle complications pre-HSCT were more likely to experience persistent pain post-HSCT.[24]

Although HLA-matched sibling transplantation has been very successful for adults and children, most patients with SCD do not have an HLA-matched sibling.[97] Alternative donor options include haploidentical, unrelated umbilical cord blood, and matched unrelated donors, most promising of which is haploidentical family members (a treatment strategy under consideration for case 1).[92] Another experimental option is gene addition using the anti-sickling β-globin vector containing the HbA^{T87Q} mutation (Bluebird Bio) that recently reported encouraging results in patients with severe beta-thalassemia.[98] This treatment is still in its early stages in SCD, but preliminary reports have revealed therapeutic expression in all 7 patients in which it was tested.[99] The relative lack of toxicity of this treatment and the ability to induce one's own hematopoietic precursors ex vivo are distinct advantages when managing the older adult with SCD.

SUMMARY AND FUTURE DIRECTIONS

Therapeutic advances and improved access to health care have contributed to greater life expectancy and consequently a growing population of older adults with SCD. The older adult with SCD is likely to have multiple aging comorbidities added to the cumulative complications of a chronic disease that largely affects the central nervous, cardiopulmonary, and renal systems. A background of chronic pain and chronic anemia not only impairs activities of daily living but also potentially worsens cognitive decline and impacts every component of their health care management and delivery. The older adult with SCD tends to have a complex medication regimen that needs careful

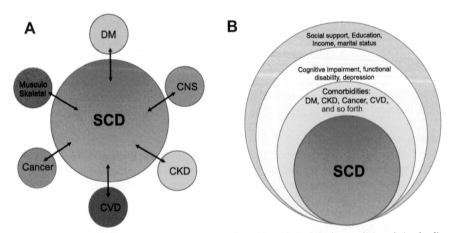

Fig. 1. A proposed model of managing SCD in the older adult. (*A*) The traditional single disease focused framework of comorbidity where comorbid conditions are considered as disease pairs, such as SCD and diabetes mellitus, SCD and cardiovascular disease, and SCD and dementia. Most clinical practice guidelines are based on this framework. (*B*) Multimorbid conceptual framework demonstrating a more patient-centric approach to managing the older adult with SCD in the context of multiple chronic conditions, geriatric syndromes, functional status, and social determinants of health. CKD, chronic kidney disease; CNS, central nervous system; CVD, cardiovascular disease; DM, diabetes mellitus.

consideration and appropriate dosage adjustments given impairment of multiple organs. Moreover, cognitive dysfunction impacts adherence requiring involvement of family members or reminders that assist in compliance with the prescribed drug regimen. The scarcity of data from clinical trials specifically aimed at treating SCD in older adults limits an evidence-based approach to treatment. In the absence of such evidence, data from randomized trials in children and younger adults with SCD are routinely extrapolated to guide management of the older adult with SCD. Thus, the basis of most management decisions for these patients reflects expert opinion or the consensus of domain experts. In recent years, great strides have been made in reducing traditional sickle-related complications, such as proteinuria, blood pressure, VTE, and cardiopulmonary disease, particularly evident in older age groups. Overall mortalities have improved, even though these are still elevated compared with adults without SCD. These trends indicate that the time has come for a fundamental shift in traditional care from single disease practices to a more patient-centered framework in a multidisciplinary team with a greater focus on geriatric conditions (**Fig. 1**).

REFERENCES

1. Williams TN, Thein SL. Sickle cell anemia and its phenotypes. Annu Rev Genomics Hum Genet 2018;19:113–47.
2. Ware RE, de Montalembert M, Tshilolo L, et al. Sickle cell disease. Lancet 2017; 390(10091):311–23.
3. Hassell KL. Population estimates of sickle cell disease in the U.S. Am J Prev Med 2010;38(4 Suppl):S512–21.
4. Hassell KL. Sickle cell disease: a continued call to action. Am J Prev Med 2016; 51(1 Suppl 1):S1–2.
5. Quinn CT, Rogers ZR, McCavit TL, et al. Improved survival of children and adolescents with sickle cell disease. Blood 2010;115(17):3447–52.
6. Telfer P, Coen P, Chakravorty S, et al. Clinical outcomes in children with sickle cell disease living in England: a neonatal cohort in East London. Haematologica 2007;92(7):905–12.
7. Paulukonis ST, Eckman JR, Snyder AB, et al. Defining sickle cell disease mortality using a population-based surveillance system, 2004 through 2008. Public Health Rep 2016;131(2):367–75.
8. Elmariah H, Garrett ME, De Castro LM, et al. Factors associated with survival in a contemporary adult sickle cell disease cohort. Am J Hematol 2014;89(5): 530–5.
9. Gardner K, Douiri A, Drasar E, et al. Survival in adults with sickle cell disease in a high-income setting. Blood 2016;128(10):1436–8.
10. Thein SL, Tisdale J. Sickle cell disease—unanswered questions and future directions in therapy. Semin Hematol 2018;55(2):51–2.
11. McGann PT, Hernandez AG, Ware RE. Sickle cell anemia in sub-Saharan Africa: advancing the clinical paradigm through partnerships and research. Blood 2017;129(2):155–61.
12. Serjeant GR, Chin N, Asnani MR, et al. Causes of death and early life determinants of survival in homozygous sickle cell disease: the Jamaican cohort study from birth. PLoS One 2018;13(3):e0192710.
13. Rees DC, Gibson JS. Biomarkers in sickle cell disease. Br J Haematol 2012; 156(4):433–45.

14. Kalpatthi R, Novelli EM. Measuring success: utility of biomarkers in sickle cell disease clinical trials and care. Hematol Am Soc Hematol Educ Program 2018;2018(1):482–92.

15. Ballas SK, Pulte ED, Lobo C, et al. Case series of octogenarians with sickle cell disease. Blood 2016;128(19):2367–9.

16. Powars DR, Chan LS, Hiti A, et al. Outcome of sickle cell anemia: a 4-decade observational study of 1056 patients. Medicine 2005;84(6):363–76.

17. Sandhu MK, Cohen A. Aging in sickle cell disease: co-morbidities and new issues in management. Hemoglobin 2015;39(4):221–4.

18. Ballas SK, Lusardi M. Hospital readmission for adult acute sickle cell painful episodes: frequency, etiology, and prognostic significance. Am J Hematol 2005; 79(1):17–25.

19. Lanzkron S, Little J, Field J, et al. Increased acute care utilization in a prospective cohort of adults with sickle cell disease. Blood Adv 2018;2(18):2412–7.

20. Panepinto JA, Brousseau DC, Hillery CA, et al. Variation in hospitalizations and hospital length of stay in children with vaso-occlusive crises in sickle cell disease. Pediatr Blood Cancer 2005;44(2):182–6.

21. Lanzkron S, Haywood C Jr. The five key things you need to know to manage adult patients with sickle cell disease. Hematol Am Soc Hematol Educ Program 2015;2015:420–5.

22. Taylor LE, Stotts NA, Humphreys J, et al. A review of the literature on the multiple dimensions of chronic pain in adults with sickle cell disease. J Pain Symptom Manage 2010;40(3):416–35.

23. Burri A, Ogata S, Rice D, et al. Twelve-year follow-up of chronic pain in twins: changes in environmental and genetic influence over time. Eur J Pain 2018. [Epub ahead of print].

24. Darbari DS, Liljencrantz J, Ikechi A, et al. Pain and opioid use after reversal of sickle cell disease following HLA-matched sibling haematopoietic stem cell transplant. Br J Haematol 2019;184(4):690–3.

25. Almeida A, Roberts I. Bone involvement in sickle cell disease. Br J Haematol 2005;129(4):482–90.

26. Milner PF, Kraus AP, Sebes JI, et al. Sickle cell disease as a cause of osteonecrosis of the femoral head. N Engl J Med 1991;325(21):1476–81.

27. Issa K, Naziri Q, Maheshwari AV, et al. Excellent results and minimal complications of total hip arthroplasty in sickle cell hemoglobinopathy at mid-term follow-up using cementless prosthetic components. J Arthroplasty 2013;28(9):1693–8.

28. Jack CM, Howard J, Aziz ES, et al. Cementless total hip replacements in sickle cell disease. Hip Int 2016;26(2):186–92.

29. Vichinsky EP, Styles LA, Colangelo LH, et al. Acute chest syndrome in sickle cell disease: clinical presentation and course. Cooperative Study of Sickle Cell Disease. Blood 1997;89(5):1787–92.

30. Castro O, Brambilla DJ, Thorington B, et al. The acute chest syndrome in sickle cell disease: incidence and risk factors. The Cooperative Study of Sickle Cell Disease. Blood 1994;84(2):643–9.

31. Vichinsky EP, Neumayr LD, Earles AN, et al. Causes and outcomes of the acute chest syndrome in sickle cell disease. National Acute Chest Syndrome Study Group. N Engl J Med 2000;342(25):1855–65.

32. Dang NC, Johnson C, Eslami-Farsani M, et al. Bone marrow embolism in sickle cell disease: a review. Am J Hematol 2005;79(1):61–7.

33. Khan AB, Kesse-Adu R, Breen C, et al. A descriptive study of the characteristics of older adults with sickle cell disease. Am J Hematol 2018;93(2):E38–40.

34. Sharma S, Efird JT, Knupp C, et al. Sleep disorders in adult sickle cell patients. J Clin Sleep Med 2015;11(3):219–23.
35. Parent F, Bachir D, Inamo J, et al. A hemodynamic study of pulmonary hypertension in sickle cell disease. N Engl J Med 2011;365(1):44–53.
36. Fonseca GH, Souza R, Salemi VM, et al. Pulmonary hypertension diagnosed by right heart catheterisation in sickle cell disease. Eur Respir J 2012;39(1):112–8.
37. Mehari A, Gladwin MT, Tian X, et al. Mortality in adults with sickle cell disease and pulmonary hypertension. JAMA 2012;307(12):1254–6.
38. Gordeuk VR, Castro OL, Machado RF. Pathophysiology and treatment of pulmonary hypertension in sickle cell disease. Blood 2016;127(7):820–8.
39. Mushemi-Blake S, Melikian N, Drasar E, et al. Pulmonary haemodynamics in sickle cell disease are driven predominantly by a high-output state rather than elevated pulmonary vascular resistance: a prospective 3-dimensional echocardiography/Doppler study. PLoS One 2015;10(8):e0135472.
40. Naik RP, Streiff MB, Haywood C Jr, et al. Venous thromboembolism incidence in the cooperative study of sickle cell disease. J Thromb Haemost 2014;12(12): 2010–6.
41. Brunson A, Lei A, Rosenberg AS, et al. Increased incidence of VTE in sickle cell disease patients: risk factors, recurrence and impact on mortality. Br J Haematol 2017;178(2):319–26.
42. Shet AS, Wun T. How I diagnose and treat venous thromboembolism in sickle cell disease. Blood 2018;132(17):1761–9.
43. Mekontso Dessap A, Deux JF, Abidi N, et al. Pulmonary artery thrombosis during acute chest syndrome in sickle cell disease. Am J Respir Crit Care Med 2011;184(9):1022–9.
44. Witt DM, Nieuwlaat R, Clark NP, et al. American Society of Hematology 2018 guidelines for management of venous thromboembolism: optimal management of anticoagulation therapy. Blood Adv 2018;2(22):3257–91.
45. Day TG, Drašar ER, Fulford T, et al. Association between hemolysis and albuminuria in adults with sickle cell anemia. Haematologica 2012;97(2):201–5.
46. Drawz P, Ayyappan S, Nouraie M, et al. Kidney disease among patients with sickle cell disease, hemoglobin SS and SC. Clin J Am Soc Nephrol 2016; 11(2):207–15.
47. Serjeant GR, Serjeant BE, Mason KP, et al. The changing face of homozygous sickle cell disease: 102 patients over 60 years. Int J Lab Hematol 2009;31(6): 585–96.
48. Sharpe CC, Thein SL. How I treat renal complications in sickle cell disease. Blood 2014;123(24):3720–6.
49. Aoki RY, Saad ST. Enalapril reduces the albuminuria of patients with sickle cell disease. Am J Med 1995;98(5):432–5.
50. Falk RJ, Scheinman J, Phillips G, et al. Prevalence and pathologic features of sickle cell nephropathy and response to inhibition of angiotensin-converting enzyme. N Engl J Med 1992;326(14):910–5.
51. Laurin LP, Nachman PH, Desai PC, et al. Hydroxyurea is associated with lower prevalence of albuminuria in adults with sickle cell disease. Nephrol Dial Transplant 2014;29(6):1211–8.
52. Steinberg MH. Erythropoietin for anemia of renal failure in sickle cell disease. N Engl J Med 1991;324(19):1369–70.
53. Berry PA, Cross TJ, Thein SL, et al. Hepatic dysfunction in sickle cell disease: a new system of classification based on global assessment. Clin Gastroenterol Hepatol 2007;5(12):1469–76 [quiz: 1369].

54. Drasar E, Igbineweka N, Vasavda N, et al. Blood transfusion usage among adults with sickle cell disease—a single institution experience over ten years. Br J Haematol 2011;152(6):766–70.

55. Ohene-Frempong K, Weiner SJ, Sleeper LA, et al. Cerebrovascular accidents in sickle cell disease: rates and risk factors. Blood 1998;91(1):288–94.

56. Birkeland P, Gardner K, Kesse-Adu R, et al. Intracranial aneurysms in sickle-cell disease are associated with the hemoglobin SS genotype but not with Moyamoya syndrome. Stroke 2016;47(7):1710–3.

57. Nabavizadeh SA, Vossough A, Ichord RN, et al. Intracranial aneurysms in sickle cell anemia: clinical and imaging findings. J Neurointerv Surg 2016;8(4):434–40.

58. Kassim AA, Pruthi S, Day M, et al. Silent cerebral infarcts and cerebral aneurysms are prevalent in adults with sickle cell anemia. Blood 2016;127(16):2038–40.

59. Vermeer SE, Prins ND, den Heijer T, et al. Silent brain infarcts and the risk of dementia and cognitive decline. N Engl J Med 2003;348(13):1215–22.

60. National Institutes of Health: National Heart Lung and Blood Institute. Evidence-based management of sickle cell disease. In: NIH expert panel report. Bethesda (MD): U.S Department of Health and Human Services; 2014. Available at: http://www.nhlbi.nih.gov/sites/www.nhlbi.nih.gov/files/sickle-cell-disease-report.pdf.

61. Yawn BP, Buchanan GR, Afenyi-Annan AN, et al. Management of sickle cell disease: summary of the 2014 evidence-based report by expert panel members. JAMA 2014;312(10):1033–48.

62. Savage WJ, Buchanan GR, Yawn BP, et al. Evidence gaps in the management of sickle cell disease: a summary of needed research. Am J Hematol 2015;90(4):273–5.

63. Charache S, Terrin ML, Moore RD, et al. Effect of hydroxyurea on the frequency of painful crises in sickle cell anemia. Investigators of the Multicenter Study of Hydroxyurea in Sickle Cell Anemia. N Engl J Med 1995;332(20):1317–22.

64. Steinberg MH, McCarthy WF, Castro O, et al. The risks and benefits of long-term use of hydroxyurea in sickle cell anemia: a 17.5 year follow-up. Am J Hematol 2010;85(6):403–8.

65. Voskaridou E, Christoulas D, Bilalis A, et al. The effect of prolonged administration of hydroxyurea on morbidity and mortality in adult patients with sickle cell syndromes: results of a 17-year, single-center trial (LaSHS). Blood 2010;115(12):2354–63.

66. Opoka RO, Ndugwa CM, Latham TS, et al. Novel use of Hydroxyurea in an African Region with Malaria (NOHARM): a trial for children with sickle cell anemia. Blood 2017;130(24):2585–93.

67. Tshilolo L, Tomlinson G, Williams TN, et al. Hydroxyurea for children with sickle cell anemia in sub-saharan Africa. N Engl J Med 2019;380(2):121–31.

68. Ballas SK, Kesen MR, Goldberg MF, et al. Beyond the definitions of the phenotypic complications of sickle cell disease: an update on management. ScientificWorldJournal 2012;2012:949535.

69. Chou ST, Fasano RM. Management of patients with sickle cell disease using transfusion therapy: guidelines and complications. Hematol Oncol Clin North Am 2016;30(3):591–608.

70. Chou ST. Transfusion therapy for sickle cell disease: a balancing act. Hematol Am Soc Hematol Educ Program 2013;2013:439–46.

71. Vichinsky EP, Earles A, Johnson RA, et al. Alloimmunization in sickle cell anemia and transfusion of racially unmatched blood. N Engl J Med 1990;322(23): 1617–21.

72. O'Suoji C, Liem RI, Mack AK, et al. Alloimmunization in sickle cell anemia in the era of extended red cell typing. Pediatr Blood Cancer 2013;60(9):1487–91.

73. Chou ST, Jackson T, Vege S, et al. High prevalence of red blood cell alloimmunization in sickle cell disease despite transfusion from Rh-matched minority donors. Blood 2013;122(6):1062–71.

74. Vidler JB, Gardner K, Amenyah K, et al. Delayed haemolytic transfusion reaction in adults with sickle cell disease: a 5-year experience. Br J Haematol 2015; 169(5):746–53.

75. de Montalembert M, Dumont MD, Heilbronner C, et al. Delayed hemolytic transfusion reaction in children with sickle cell disease. Haematologica 2011;96(6): 801–7.

76. Pirenne F, Yazdanbakhsh K. How I safely transfuse patients with sickle-cell disease and manage delayed hemolytic transfusion reactions. Blood 2018;131(25): 2773–81.

77. Chou ST, Evans P, Vege S, et al. RH genotype matching for transfusion support in sickle cell disease. Blood 2018;132(11):1198–207.

78. Hendrickson JE, Tormey CA, Shaz BH. Red blood cell alloimmunization mitigation strategies. Transfus Med Rev 2014;28(3):137–44.

79. Hendrickson JE, Tormey CA. Rhesus pieces: genotype matching of RBCs. Blood 2018;132(11):1091–3.

80. Drasar E, Vasavda N, Igbineweka N, et al. Serum ferritin and total units transfused for assessing iron overload in adults with sickle cell disease. Br J Haematol 2012;157(5):645–7.

81. Porter J, Garbowski M. Consequences and management of iron overload in sickle cell disease. Hematol Am Soc Hematol Educ Program 2013;2013:447–56.

82. St Pierre TG, Clark PR, Chua-anusorn W, et al. Non-invasive measurement and imaging of liver iron concentrations using proton magnetic resonance. Blood 2005;105(2):855–61.

83. Davis BA, Allard S, Qureshi A, et al. Guidelines on red cell transfusion in sickle cell disease. Part I: principles and laboratory aspects. Br J Haematol 2017; 176(2):179–91.

84. Davis BA, Allard S, Qureshi A, et al. Guidelines on red cell transfusion in sickle cell disease Part II: indications for transfusion. Br J Haematol 2017;176(2): 192–209.

85. Niihara Y, Miller ST, Kanter J, et al. A phase 3 trial of l-glutamine in sickle cell disease. N Engl J Med 2018;379(3):226–35.

86. Ataga KI, Kutlar A, Kanter J, et al. Crizanlizumab for the prevention of pain crises in sickle cell disease. N Engl J Med 2017;376(5):429–39.

87. Blyden G, Bridges KR, Bronte L. Case series of patients with severe sickle cell disease treated with voxelotor (GBT440) by compassionate access. Am J Hematol 2018. [Epub ahead of print].

88. Telen MJ, Wun T, McCavit TL, et al. Randomized phase 2 study of GMI-1070 in SCD: reduction in time to resolution of vaso-occlusive events and decreased opioid use. Blood 2015;125(17):2656–64.

89. Molokie R, Lavelle D, Gowhari M, et al. Oral tetrahydrouridine and decitabine for non-cytotoxic epigenetic gene regulation in sickle cell disease: a randomized phase 1 study. PLoS Med 2017;14(9):e1002382.

90. Lavelle D, Engel JD, Saunthararajah Y. Fetal hemoglobin induction by epigenetic drugs. Semin Hematol 2018;55(2):60–7.

91. Guilcher GMT, Truong TH, Saraf SL, et al. Curative therapies: allogeneic hematopoietic cell transplantation from matched related donors using myeloablative, reduced intensity, and nonmyeloablative conditioning in sickle cell disease. Semin Hematol 2018;55(2):87–93.

92. Joseph JJ, Abraham AA, Fitzhugh CD. When there is no match, the game is not over: alternative donor options for hematopoietic stem cell transplantation in sickle cell disease. Semin Hematol 2018;55(2):94–101.

93. Esrick EB, Bauer DE. Genetic therapies for sickle cell disease. Semin Hematol 2018;55(2):76–86.

94. Gluckman E, Cappelli B, Bernaudin F, et al. Sickle cell disease: an international survey of results of HLA-identical sibling hematopoietic stem cell transplantation. Blood 2017;129(11):1548–56.

95. Fitzhugh CD, Walters MC. The case for HLA-identical sibling hematopoietic stem cell transplantation in children with symptomatic sickle cell anemia. Blood Adv 2017;1(26):2563–7.

96. Hsieh MM, Fitzhugh CD, Weitzel RP, et al. Nonmyeloablative HLA-matched sibling allogeneic hematopoietic stem cell transplantation for severe sickle cell phenotype. JAMA 2014;312(1):48–56.

97. Walters MC, De Castro LM, Sullivan KM, et al. Indications and results of HLA-identical sibling hematopoietic cell transplantation for sickle cell disease. Biol Blood Marrow Transplant 2016;22(2):207–11.

98. Thompson AA, Walters MC, Kwiatkowski J, et al. Gene therapy in patients with transfusion-dependent beta-thalassemia. N Engl J Med 2018;378(16):1479–93.

99. Ribeil JA, Hacein-Bey-Abina S, Payen E, et al. Gene therapy in a patient with sickle cell disease. N Engl J Med 2017;376(9):848–55.

100. Smith WR, Penberthy LT, Bovbjerg VE, et al. Daily assessment of pain in adults with sickle cell disease. Ann Intern Med 2008;148(2):94–101.

101. Smith WR, McClish DK, Dahman BA, et al. Daily home opioid use in adults with sickle cell disease: the PiSCES project. J Opioid Manag 2015;11(3):243–53.

102. Gladwin MT, Sachdev V, Jison ML, et al. Pulmonary hypertension as a risk factor for death in patients with sickle cell disease. N Engl J Med 2004;350(9):886–95.

103. Gladwin MT, Barst RJ, Gibbs JS, et al. Risk factors for death in 632 patients with sickle cell disease in the United States and United Kingdom. PLoS One 2014; 9(7):e99489.

104. Klings ES, Wyszynski DF, Nolan VG, et al. Abnormal pulmonary function in adults with sickle cell anemia. Am J Respir Crit Care Med 2006;173(11):1264–9.

105. DeBaun MR, Kirkham FJ. Central nervous system complications and management in sickle cell disease. Blood 2016;127(7):829–38.

106. Strouse JJ, Jordan LC, Lanzkron S, et al. The excess burden of stroke in hospitalized adults with sickle cell disease. Am J Hematol 2009;84(9):548–52.

107. Adeyoju AB, Olujohungbe AB, Morris J, et al. Priapism in sickle-cell disease; incidence, risk factors and complications—an international multicentre study. BJU Int 2002;90(9):898–902.

108. Hernigou P, Habibi A, Bachir D, et al. The natural history of asymptomatic osteonecrosis of the femoral head in adults with sickle cell disease. J Bone Joint Surg Am 2006;88(12):2565–72.

109. Serjeant GR. Leg ulceration in sickle cell anemia. Arch Intern Med 1974;133(4): 690–4.

110. Koshy M, Entsuah R, Koranda A, et al. Leg ulcers in patients with sickle cell disease. Blood 1989;74(4):1403–8.
111. Vasavda N, Menzel S, Kondaveeti S, et al. The linear effects of alpha-thalassaemia, the UGT1A1 and HMOX1 polymorphisms on cholelithiasis in sickle cell disease. Br J Haematol 2007;138(2):263–70.
112. Mathew R, Bafiq R, Ramu J, et al. Spectral domain optical coherence tomography in patients with sickle cell disease. Br J Ophthalmol 2015;99(7):967–72.
113. Downes SM, Hambleton IR, Chuang EL, et al. Incidence and natural history of proliferative sickle cell retinopathy: observations from a cohort study. Ophthalmology 2005;112(11):1869–75.

Heyde Syndrome
Aortic Stenosis and Beyond

Joseph L. Blackshear, MD

KEYWORDS

- von Willebrand factor • Heyde syndrome • Aortic stenosis • Angiodysplasia
- Gastrointestinal bleeding • Acquired von Willebrand syndrome

KEY POINTS

- Bleeding may accompany valvular heart disease, hypertrophic cardiomyopathy, and left ventricular assist device (LVAD) therapy.
- Most patients with moderate or greater cardiac lesions demonstrate laboratory findings consistent with acquired von Willebrand syndrome (AVWS).
- Gastrointestinal angiodysplasia has been associated with congenital and AVWS.
- Laboratory tests for AVWS include platelet function analyzer 100, von Willebrand factor (VWF) antigen and activity, and VWF multimer analysis.
- Severe gastrointestinal bleeding in AVWS due to cardiac disorders often recurs after endoscopic treatment but responds to cardiac repair, with normalization of VWF function.

 Video content accompanies this article at http://www.geriatric.theclinics.com.

INTRODUCTION

Monomers of von Willebrand factor (VWF) are synthesized in the ribosomes of endothelial cells and platelets, dimerized in the endoplasmic reticulum, and, in the golgi, multimers of as many as 20 monomers to 40 monomers are constructed. After ultra-large multimers are secreted into plasma, strands are elongated in the microcirculation and undergo proteolysis by ADAMTS13. Presecretion forms contain 20 to 40 monomers whereas mature circulating forms consist of 2 to 25 monomers. Multimers greater than 10 monomers are hemostatically effective but comprise only 4% of total protein. Half of VWF is 5 monomer units or smaller.[1–4] Remultimerization does not occur after release into plasma, and, therefore, shortened VWF suggests the presence of the lesion and its severity. VWF also regulates angiogenesis, suggesting a link between VWF and thus the association of intestinal angiodysplasia.[5,6] Cardiac lesions elongate VWF multimers in the shear field, resulting in proteolytic loss of the highest

Disclosure statement: The author has nothing to disclose.
Department of Cardiovascular Diseases, Mayo Clinic Florida, 4500 San Pablo Road, Jacksonville, FL 32224, USA
E-mail address: blackshear.joseph@mayo.edu

molecular weight forms, as is shown in a patient with an obstructed aortic prosthesis (**Fig. 1**, Videos 1 and 2).

Analysis of VWF multimers is central to the diagnosis of Heyde syndrome. To compare the severity of disruption of VWF, the author and others have reported a normalized multimer ratio, as shown in **Fig. 1**. Plasma from normal controls yields a value of 1.0 and between 0.40 and 0.50 for patients with extreme VWF dysfunction, such as with left ventricular assist devices (LVADs). In a real-world demonstration of the utility, the normalized multimer ratio showed little change after aortic valvuloplasty for severe aortic stenosis, a technique known to produce only a modest change in gradient, whereas valve replacement corrected the ratio to normal.[7] Values in recent articles[7-9] are essentially identical to values reported in 1980 by Weinstein and colleagues.[10]

The platelet function analyzer (PFA) closure time—normal, less than 121 seconds; abnormal, 121 seconds to 300 seconds; and nonclotting, greater than or equal to 300 seconds—is point-of-care, recognized screening test for von Willebrand diseases.[11,12] It has the advantage of immediate results, as opposed to a week turnaround for VWF multimers. With the most severe loss of VWF function, as with LVAD, very severe aortic stenosis, or obstructive hypertrophic cardiomyopathy, a majority of samples of PFA do not clot during the 300-second testing period. Ratios of either VWF activity or VWF collagen binding activity to antigen are used but are less sensitive than either VWF multimers or PFA.[9]

ACQUIRED VON WILLEBRAND SYNDROME, BROADLY

In **Table 1**, the recognized etiologies of acquired von Willebrand syndrome (AVWS) are listed.[13,14] From a registry initially published in 2000, reported cases suggested that

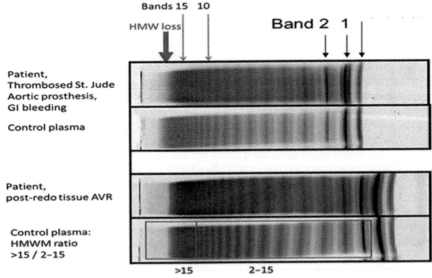

Fig. 1. Gel electrophoresis of VWF in a patient with a thrombosed mechanical heart valve, high gradient, and gastrointestinal hemorrhage (see Videos 1 and 2). Note the loss of multimers with repeat units greater than approximately 18, which recovered after redo valve replacement surgery. At the bottom, an illustration of the greater than 15/2 to 15 multimer ratio is shown. The normalized multimer ratio consists of this ratio in the patient divided by the ratio of control plasma. AVR, aortic valve replacement; GI, gastrointestinal; HMW, high molecular weight; HMWM, high molecular weight multimer.

Table 1	
Acquired von Willebrand syndrome	
Category (Percentage of All Acquired von Willebrand Syndrome)	Disease or Association
Shear-induced (ADAMTS13) (21%)	Aortic stenosis, hypertrophic obstructive cardiomyopathy, VSD, LVAD, pulmonary hypertension
Thrombocytosis (marked) and proteolysis (15%)	Essential thrombocythemia, other myeloproliferative neoplasms
Antibodies to VWF (48%)	Monoclonal gammopathies: autoimmune disease, lymphoproliferative disorders
Aberrant VWF binding to tumor cells (5%)	Wilms tumor, certain plasma cell disorders (in some cases to aberrantly expressed glycoprotein 1b)
Decreased VWF synthesis	Hypothyroidism
Drug related	Ciprofloxacin, valproic acid, griseofulvin, hydroxyethyl starch

Data from Federici AB, Rand JH, Buciarelli P, et al. Acquired von Willebrand syndrome: data from an international registry. Thromb Haemostasis 2000;84:345–9; and Nichols WL, Rick ME, Ortel TL, et al. Clinical and laboratory diagnosis of von Willebrand disease: a synopsis of the 2008 NHLBI/NIH guidelines. Am J Hematol 2009;84:366–70.

hematologic entities were more common than cardiovascular causes, but subsequent reports[1] have argued that the opposite is true, and a new Web-interactive registry of cases is being compiled, where readers may enter their own cases at www.intreavws.com. Although the term, Heyde syndrome, is specific for aortic stenosis and bleeding from AVWS, the same mechanism has been implicated in disorders with high intravascular shear; thus, any of these entities is regarded as constituting Heyde syndrome in this article. Because aortic stenosis is present in 7.5% of persons age 75 or greater, whereas monoclonal gammopathy of uncertain significance is present in 6.6% of white persons older than 80 years, it is thus possible for both disorders to exist in the same person. **Fig. 2** illustrates such a case and demonstrates the key differences in VWF multimer pattern in the 2 pathophysiologies.

AORTIC STENOSIS, THE HISTORY AND THE PRESENT

- 1958: Heyde described "at least 10 patients with calcific aortic stenosis who had massive gastrointestinal (GI) bleeding for which we could discover no cause."
- 1974, 1980: association with gastrointestinal angiodysplasia suggested[15,16]
- 1986: decreased high-molecular-weight multimers suggested by Gill[17]
- 1987: nearly all patients with Heyde syndrome treated for bleeding recurred, whereas 94% who had aortic valve replacement were cured[18]
- 1992: Warkentin[19] puts forth the hypothesis that the syndrome is linked to VWF.
- 2003: Vincentelli and colleagues[20] report aortic stenosis patients before and after surgery with data, including multimers, PFA, and VWF collagen binding to VWF antigen ratios.
- 2006: heart failure guideline publication states: "In patients with severe [aortic stenosis] AS, AVWS is associated with clinical bleeding in approximately 20% of patients, and resolves after aortic valve replacement."
- 2012: Thompson and colleagues[21] report that aortic valve replacement was curative of bleeding in 79% of patients.

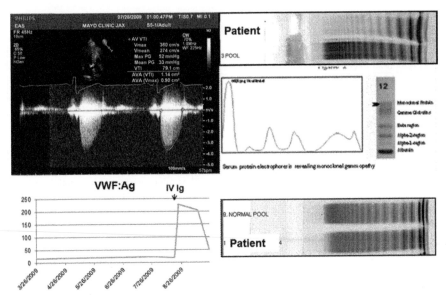

Fig. 2. A 90-year-old man with aortic stenosis (peak velocity 3.5 m/s = moderate aortic stenosis [*upper left*]) had recurrent gastrointestinal bleeding with angiodysplasias. Cardiac surgery was considered. VWF antigen, however, was markedly reduced, at 8% (normal ≥70%), and VWF multimer analysis revealed marked reduction of most multimers (*upper right*). This pattern is not typical for severe aortic stenosis, in which VWF antigen should be normal, and high-molecular-weight multimers should be reduced. Protein electrophoresis revealed monoclonal protein of undetermined significance (*middle right*); treatment with intravenous immunoglobulin stopped bleeding and increased VWF antigen level (*lower left*); and the VWF multimer pattern corrected to a typical pattern for aortic stenosis (*lower right*).

Prevalence for bleeding in patients with aortic stenosis between 7% and 20% has been published.[9,22–25] Different investigators, however, required more restrictive definitions and reported figures as low as 2%.[26,27] Nonetheless, because aortic stenosis is common and increasing in frequency in the United States as life expectancy is prolonged, the number of Heyde syndrome patients likely will increase in coming years.

LEFT VENTRICULAR ASSIST DEVICE PATIENTS

All continuous-flow LVAD patients have loss of high-molecular-weight VWF multimers, compared with 71% to 80% in severe aortic stenosis. Gastrointestinal bleeding complicates modern LVAD therapy in 20% to 40% of patients, and angiodysplasia has been the most common lesion found at endoscopy.[28] Patients with LVAD and bleeding who undergo cardiac transplantation and LVAD removal are cured of gastrointestinal hemorrhage. The approach to management of the bleeding LVAD patient is an important and highly risky and complex affair, because reduction in anticoagulant intensity is often an initial step but one that also increases the risk of pump thrombosis and stroke.

Re-engineering of devices may be able to mitigate this problem to some extent. The author's group compared patients implanted with a high rotational speed LVAD, usual revolutions per minute (RPMs) 9500, to a device with usual rotational speeds of 2600 RPMs. VWF normalized multimer ratios trended in the direction of less severely abnormal multimers, with the lower versus the higher speed device in this small study (**Fig. 3**).

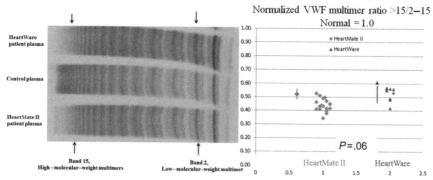

Fig. 3. Comparison of normalized multimer ratios in LVAD with lower rotational speed (HeartWare) and higher rotational speed (HeartMate II). (*Data from* Gupta BP, Leoni J, Patel P, et al. Blood 2015;126:2306.)

Another group evaluated a next-generation device designed for improved hemo-compatibility with a magnetically levitated device rotor, allowing a wider flow path. Significantly less degradation of high-molecular-weight multimers was found in the newer device versus the high-speed comparator.[29]

AORTIC REGURGITATION

VWF multimer data in patients undergoing aortic valve replacement for severe aortic insufficiency were first reported in 9 patients by Weinstein and colleagues[10] in 1980. Budde and colleagues[30] reported AVWS with gastrointestinal bleeding in 2 patients with aortic regurgitation from endocarditis. Wan and colleagues[31] reported a similar case in a patient who also had longstanding mitral regurgitation. The author's group has published data from patients with varying degrees of native aortic insufficiency and found that VWF multimers were abnormal in the great majority of patients with moderate to severe aortic regurgitation but not mild aortic regurgitation (**Fig. 4**). By comparisons of the normalized multimer ratio, the degree of abnormality was less than in aortic stenosis or mitral regurgitation.[32] Two of the 21 patients with moderate to severe aortic regurgitation had a history of gastrointestinal bleeding. Severe isolated native aortic regurgitation is less common than either aortic stenosis or mitral regurgitation. Overall, although Heyde syndrome has rarely been reported in native aortic insufficiency, as discussed, it does occur with frequency in patients with regurgitation from aortic prosthetic valves.

MITRAL REGURGITATION

There have been hints over several years that Heyde syndrome may exist in mitral regurgitation:

- 1981: Pickering and colleagues[33] described 15 patients with von Willebrand disease, 8 of whom had mitral regurgitation due to mitral valve prolapse.
- 1988: Weinstein and colleagues[10] described loss of VWF high-molecular-weight multimers, which resolved after surgery in 10 patients with mitral regurgitation.
- 2002: Budde and colleagues[30] reported 2 patients with endocarditis associated mitral regurgitation with bleeding and AVWS.
- 2005: Tarnow and colleagues[34] described abnormal VWF multimers in Cavalier King Charles spaniels with myxomatous mitral valves, cardiac murmurs, and a bleeding tendency.

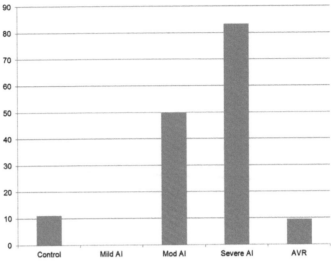

Fig. 4. Frequency of abnormal VWF multimers in native aortic regurgitation. PFA-100 closure times (normal <121 seconds) were concordant with (mean, range) values for mild (86, 62–100), mild to moderate (142, 100–300), and moderate to severe (163, 83–300) respectively. AI, aortic insufficiency; AVR, aortic valve replacement.

After encountering patients with severe mitral regurgitation and gastrointestinal bleeding from intestinal angiodysplasia who had been referred to the author's institution for double-balloon enteroscopy (**Fig. 5**, Videos 3 and 4), the authors sought to systematically define VWF function in similar patients (n = 53).[35] A strong correlation of the severity of mitral regurgitation to the degree of VWF multimer loss was noted, and similar findings were found for PFA testing and the ratio of VWF activity to antigen. Clinically important bleeding was noted in 9 patients, and 7 had intestinal angiodysplasia and transfusion-dependent gastrointestinal bleeding, with median (interquartile range) number of transfusions required 20, range 4 to 50. In patients who underwent mitral valve repair or replacement (n = 20), all measures of VWF function improved. Thus, as with aortic stenosis, the turbulence associated with moderate to severe mitral regurgitation is sufficient to produce abnormalities in VWF activity in most patients. AVWS-related bleeding may occur, and the syndrome is reversible with mitral valve surgery.

HYPERTROPHIC CARDIOMYOPATHY

Hypertrophic cardiomyopathy, gastrointestinal hemorrhage, and angiodysplasia have been case reported sporadically in the past, and relief from bleeding was reported with definitive pressure gradient–reducing therapies. A single case report identified loss of high-molecular-weight multimers of VWF, with some improvement after intensification of medical therapy (case reports reviewed in references[36,37]). LeTourneau and colleagues[38] in 2008 described 28 patients who had subaortic obstruction. Loss of high-molecular-weight multimers of VWF correlated to the magnitude of left ventricular outflow obstruction. The author first encountered a patient with hypertrophic cardiomyopathy and Heyde syndrome bleeding in 2006, and subsequently reported

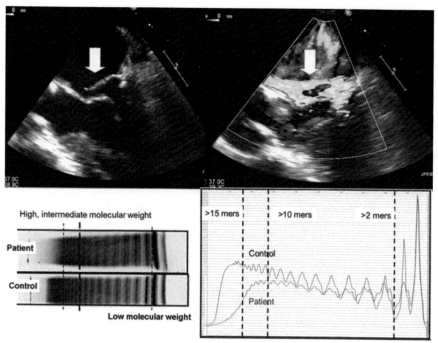

Fig. 5. An 85-year-old man had transfusion-dependent gastrointestinal bleeding and small bowel angiodysplasia. Physical examination revealed a grade IV/VI systolic murmur. Echocardiography documented a flail mitral valve posterior leaflet (*top left*) and severe regurgitation (*top right arrows*). PFA-100 collagen-adenosine closure time was 221 seconds (normal <121 seconds). VWF gel electrophoresis showed loss of high-molecular-weight to low-intermediate weight multimers (*bottom left*). Denistometric analysis of VWF gel (*bottom right*). The patient was offered surgical repair but declined.

"cure" from surgical septal myectomy in this first patient and 4 others in 2011. The author subsequently studied additional patients[37,39] and found the following:

- Multiple tests of VWF function reflected the severity of the outflow tract gradient.
- The degree of dysfunction of VWF by multiple tests was nearly as severe as in LVAD.
- Septal myectomy normalized VWF multimers whereas other therapies were less effective.
- Bleeding resolved with septal reduction therapy.

There are important demographic findings in these patients. Although the first patient from the author's 2011 series was a man, the 4 additional cases in that initial report, and all 11 cases with transfusion dependence in a subsequent report, were elderly women.[37] Non–transfusion-dependent gastrointestinal bleeding and other bleeding occurred in men and women, and epistaxis was a frequent finding. Although the author's studies suffer from referral bias, an overall prevalence of abnormal bleeding was found in 26% of patients with hypertrophic cardiomyopathy. Bleeding was more likely with advancing age and female gender.

MITRAL PROSTHESIS DYSFUNCTION

In 2011, Perez-Rodriguez and colleagues[40] reported 5 cases of bleeding with abnormal VWF multimers in patients with mitral paravalvular leak. Bleeding and

VWF multimers normalized after surgical repair of the paravalvular leak. The author studied normally functioning mitral valve replacement or repair patients in comparison to dysfunctional mitral replacement or repair (**Table 2**).[32] There were marked differences in VWF function between normal and dysfunctional valves. Gastrointestinal bleeding was found in 5 of 19 patients with dysfunctional mitral replacement or repair. Some of the patients have been treated with percutaneous plug insertion for paravalvular leak but there are insufficient data to determine whether or not bleeding or the severity of VWF abnormalities consistently improves.

SURGICAL AND TRANSCATHETER AORTIC PROSTHESIS DYSFUNCTION

Thrombosis in mechanical as well as tissue valves[41] is one of several mechanisms of prosthesis dysfunction, which also includes degenerative calcification and obstruction, central valve leakage, leaflet tear, and paravalvular regurgitation. This issue is of extreme importance because tissue valve replacement is done in the aortic valve in 85% of patients, and all tissue valves eventually fail, usually between 7 years and 20 years. It, therefore, is possible that a patient with prior aortic stenosis may develop either recurrent aortic stenosis or new aortic regurgitation and have recurrent bleeding.

The author's group evaluated 24 surgical or transcatheter aortic valve implants with prosthesis dysfunction. Gastrointestinal bleeding and laboratory evidence of VWF dysfunction were far more common in dysfunctional valves in comparison to normally functioning aortic valve implants (see **Table 2**).[32] Similarly, Spangenberg and colleagues[42] found abnormal VWF function in 2 transcatheter aortic valve implant patients with moderate to severe paravalvular regurgitation as did Van Belle and colleagues[8] in 4 patients. Genereaux and colleagues[43] reported late major bleeding after transcatheter aortic valve replacement in 5.9% of patients. Gastrointestinal bleeding was the most common type of late bleeding and moderate to severe paravalvular leak was an independent predictor of late major bleeding. VWF testing was not performed.

Van Belle and colleagues[8] studied quantitative VWF multimers and PFA testing in the setting of transcatheter aortic valve implantation for aortic stenosis. PFA corrected in patients who had no or mild paravalvular regurgitation postprocedure but did not correct in patients who had greater than or equal to moderate aortic regurgitation after catheter valve deployment. Persistent abnormalities of PFA noted during the procedure with greater than or equal to moderate aortic regurgitation prompted repeat attempts to dilate catheter implanted valves and corrected abnormal multimers in 20 of 46 valves.

Table 2
Comparative von Willebrand factor findings in normal versus dysfunctional aortic or mitral valve prostheses

Prosthetic Valve Type	n	Abnormal Multimer	Platelet Function Analyzer 100 Mean	Heyde Syndrome
Normal aortic prosthesis	26	1 (4%)	108	0
Greater than or equal to moderate AO prosthesis dysfunction	24	20 (83%)	157	6 (25%)
Normal mitral valve prosthesis or repair	36	2 (6%)	91	0
Greater than or equal to moderate mitral prosthesis dysfunction	19	14 (74%)	159	5 (26%)

CLINICAL APPROACH TO THE PATIENT AND REMAINING UNKNOWNS

Patients with obscure recurrent gastrointestinal bleeding usually undergo an initial endoscopic assessment, and the author's approach is to advise panendoscopy at least once to ensure that a tumor or other nonangiodysplasia bleeding source is not missed. Angiodysplasias are difficult to find, and in a patient with a cardiac lesion with normal endoscopy or showing angiodysplasia, the author next proceeds to comprehensive echocardiographic evaluation, usually with both transthoracic and transesophageal echocardiography. A VWF panel, including VWF activity, antigen, and multimers, and PFA testing, is performed. Cardiac repair is a strong consideration for patients with moderate to severe cardiac lesions and transfusion-dependent bleeding and laboratory evidence of AVWS.

It remains uncertain why all LVAD patients, and most patients with moderate to severe cardiac lesions, have abnormal VWF testing, but clinical bleeding and intestinal angiodyplasia occur in only a subset of these. The fragment from degraded VWF, which signals intestinal epithelium to produce angiodysplasia, also remains undefined. Finally, nonsurgical approaches to some cardiac lesions, such as mitral valve percutaneous clip repair and transcatheter paravalvular leak plugging, are used for refractory heart failure symptoms. Compared with surgical repair, there is less hemodynamic resolution of valve or prosthesis dysfunction, and it is unclear if these procedures can improve VWF function enough to stop bleeding in any individual with Heyde syndrome from valve dysfunction.

SUPPLEMENTARY DATA

Supplementary data related to this article can be found online at https://doi.org/10.1016/j.cger.2019.03.007.

REFERENCES

1. Tiede A, Priesack J, Sersitzke S, et al. Diagnostic workup of patients with acquired von Willebrand syndrome: a retrospective single-center cohort study. J Thromb Haemost 2008;6:569–76.
2. Studt JD, Budde U, Schneppenheim R, et al. Quantification and facilitated comparison of von Willebrand factor multimer patterns by densitometry. Am J Clin Pathol 2001;116(4):567–74.
3. Lippok S, Obser T, Muller JP, et al. Exponential size distribution of von Willebrand factor. Biophys J 2013;105:1208–16.
4. Lenting P, Casari C, Christophe OD, et al. von Willebrand factor: the old, the new, and the unknown. J Thromb Haemost 2012;10:2428–37.
5. Starke RD, Ferraro F, Paschalaki KE, et al. Endothelial von Willebrand factor regulates angiogenesis. Blood 2011;117:1071–80.
6. Franchini M, Mannucci PM. von Willebrand disease-associated angiodysplasia: a few answers, still many questions. Br J Haematol 2013;16:177–82.
7. Van Belle E, Rauch A, Vincentelli A, et al. Von Willebrand factor as a biological sensor of blood flow to monitor percutaneous aortic valve interventions. Circ Res 2015;116:1193–201.
8. Van Belle E, Rauch A, Vincent F, et al. von Willebrand factor multimers during transcatheter aortic valve replacement. N Engl J Med 2016;375:335–44.
9. Blackshear J, Wysokinska E, Safford R, et al. Indexes of von Willebrand factor as biomarkers of aortic stenosis severity (from the biomarkers of aortic stenosis severity [BASS] study). Am J Cardiol 2013;111:374–81.

10. Weinstein M, Ware JA, Troll J, et al. Changes in von Willebrand factor during cardiac surgery: effect of desmopressin acetate. Blood 1988;71:1648–55.
11. Chen YC, Yang L, Cheng SN, et al. von Willebrand disease: a clinical and laboratory study of 65 patients. Ann Hematol 2011;90:1183–90.
12. Weiss DR, Strasser DF, Ringwald J, et al. High resolution multimer analysis and the PFA-100 platelet function analyzer can detect von Willebrand disease type 2A without a patholocial ratio of ristocetin cofactor activity and von Willebrand antigen level. Clin Lab 2012;58:1203–9.
13. Federici AB, Rand JH, Buciarelli P, et al. Acquired von Willebrand syndrome: data from an international registry. Thromb Haemost 2000;84:345–9.
14. Nichols WL, Rick ME, Ortel TL, et al. Clinical and laboratory diagnosis of von Willebrand disease: a synopsis of the 2008 NHLBI/NIH guidelines. Am J Hematol 2009;84:366–70.
15. Cody MC, O'Donovan TP, Hughes RW Jr. Idiopathic gastrointestinal bleeding and aortic stenosis. Am J Dig Dis 1974;19:393–8.
16. Roges BH. Endoscopic diagnosis and therapy on mucosal vascular abnormalities of the gastrointestinal tract occurring in elderly patients and associated with cardiac, vascular, and pulmonary disease. Gastrointest Endosc 1980;26: 134–8.
17. Gill JC, Wilson AD, Endres-Brooks J, et al. Loss of the largest von Willebrand factor multimers from the plasma of patients with congenital cardiac defects. Blood 1986;67:758–61.
18. King RM, Pluth JR, Giuliani ER. The association of unexplained gastrointestinal bleeding with calcific aortic stenosis. Ann Thorac Surg 1987;44:514–6.
19. Warkentin TE, Moore JC, Morgan DG. Aortic stenosis and bleeding gastrointestinal angiodysplasia: is acquired von Willebrand syndrome the link? Lancet 1992;340:35–7.
20. Vincentelli A, Susen S, Le Tourneau T, et al. Acquired von Willebrand syndrome in aortic stenosis. N Engl J Med 2003;349:343–9.
21. Thompson JL, Schaff HV, Dearani JA, et al. Risk of recurrent gastrointestinal bleeding after aortic valve replacement in patients with Heyde syndrome. J Thorac Cardiovasc Surg 2012;144:112–6.
22. Yoshida K, Tobe S, Kawata M, et al. Acquired and reversible von Willebrand disease with high shear stress aortic valve stenosis. Ann Thorac Surg 2006;81: 490–4.
23. Sucker C, Feindtz P, Zotzi RB, et al. Functional von Willebrand factor assays are not predictive for the absence of highest-molecular weight von Willebrand factor multimers in patients with aortic-valve stenosis. Thromb Haemost 2005;94:465–6.
24. Casonato A, Sponga S, Pontara E. von Willbrand factor abnormalities in aortic valve stensosis: pathophysiology and impact on bleeding. Thromb Haemost 2011;106:58–66.
25. Solomon C, Budde U, Schneppenheim S. Acquired type 2A von Willebrand syndrome caused by aortic valve disease corrects during valve surgery. Br J Anaesth 2011;106:494–500.
26. Godino C, Lauretta L, Pavon AG, et al. Heyde's syndrome incidence and outcome in patients undergoing transcatheter aortic valve implantation. J Am Coll Cardiol 2013;61:687–9.
27. Caspar T, Jesel L, Desprez D, et al. Effects of transcutaneous aortic valve implantation on aortic valve disease-related hemostatic disorders involving von Willebrand factor. Can J Cardiol 2015;31:738–43.

28. Guha A, Eshelbrenner CL, Richards DM, et al. Gastrointestinal bleeding after continuous flow left ventricular device implantation: review of pathophysiology and management. Methodist Debakey Cardiovasc J 2015;11:24–7.
29. Netuka I, Kvasnicka T, Kvasnicka J, et al. Evaluation of von Willebrand factor with a fully magnetically levitated centrifugal continuous-flow left ventricular assist device in advanced heart failure. J Heart Lung Transplant 2016;35:860–7.
30. Budde U, Bergmann F, Michiels JJ. Acquired von Willebrand syndrome: experience from 2 years in a single laboratory compared with data from the literature and an international registry. Semin Thromb Hemost 2002;28:227–38.
31. Wan SH, Liang JJ, Vaidya R, et al. Acquired von Willebrand syndrome secondary to mitral and aortic regurgitation. Can J Cardiol 2014;30:1108.e9-10.
32. Blackshear JL, McRee CW, Safford RE, et al. von Willebrand factor abnormalities and heyde syndrome in dysfunctional heart valve prostheses. JAMA Cardiol 2016;1:198–204.
33. Pickering NJ, Brody JI, Barrett MJ. von Willebrand syndromes and mitral-valve prolapse – linked mesenchymal dysplasia. N Engl J Med 1981;305:131–4.
34. Tarnow I, Kristensen AT, Olsen LH, et al. Dogs with heart diseases causing turbulent high-velocity blood flow have changes in platelet function and von Willebrand factor multimer distribution. J Vet Intern Med 2005;19:515–22.
35. Blackshear JL, Wysokinska EM, Safford RE, et al. Shear stress-associated acquired von Willebrand syndrome in patients with mitral regurgitation. J Thromb Haemost 2014;12:1966–74.
36. Blackshear JL, Schaff HV, Ommen SR, et al. Hypertrophic obstructive cardiomyopathy, bleeding history, and acquired von Willebrand syndrome: response to septal myectomy. Mayo Clin Proc 2011;86:219–24.
37. Blackshear JL, Stark ME, Agnew RC, et al. Remission of recurrent gastrointestinal bleeding after septal reduction therapy in patients with hypertrophic obstructive cardiomyopathy-associated acquired von Willebrand syndrome. J Thromb Haemost 2015;13:191–6.
38. Le Tourneau TL, Susen S, Caron C, et al. Functional impairment of von Willebrand factor in hypertrophic cardiomyopathy: relation to rest and exercise obstruction. Circulation 2008;118:1550–7.
39. Blackshear JL, Kusumoto H, Safford RE, et al. Usefulness of von Willebrand factor activity indexes to predict therapeutic response in hypertrophic cardiomyopathy. Am J Cardiol 2016;117:436–42.
40. Perez-Rodriguez A, Pinto JC, Loures E, et al. Acquired von Willebrand syndrome and mitral valve prosthesis leakage. A pilot study. Eur J Haematol 2011;87:448–56.
41. Makkar RR, Fontana G, Julaihaw H, et al. Possible subclinical valve thrombosis in bioprosthetic aortic valves. N Engl J Med 2015;373:2015–24.
42. Spangenberg T, Budde U, Schewel D, et al. Loss of high molecular weight multimers of Von Willebrand factor in aortic stenosis with transcatheter aortic valve replacement (TAVR). JACC Cardiovasc Interv 2016;8:692–700.
43. Genereaux P, Cohen DJ, Mack M, et al. Incidence, predictors, and prognostic impact of late bleeding complications after transcatheter aortic valve replacement. J Am Coll Cardiol 2014;64:2605–16.

Anemia in the Long-Term Care Setting

Syed Ashad Abid, MD, MPH[a], Stefan Gravenstein, MD, MPH[a,b], Aman Nanda, MD[a,*]

KEYWORDS

- Anemia • Long-term care • Nursing home • Geriatric • Elderly • Iron deficiency

KEY POINTS

- The prevalence of anemia is high among residents living in long-term care setting.
- Anemia is associated with increased risk for falls, decline in physical performance as well as in quality of life.
- Evaluation and treatment of anemia should be based on patient's and caregiver's wishes, goals of care, and whether it will improve quality of life.

INTRODUCTION

Institutionalized elderly have multiple morbidities that are commonly associated with anemia. These conditions include cognitive impairment, frailty, renal disease, heart failure, bleeding and nutritional issues, and, like anemia, associate with a risk of falls. Recognizing the consequences of anemia can be confounded by signs and symptoms associated with comorbid conditions in older people and age-related reduction in organ functional capacity and physiologic reserve. However, the literature on anemia in long-term care settings is quite limited. Considering the potential importance of anemia on quality of life, it may be appropriate to evaluate and treat it. But which long-term care adult should be formally evaluated, and how does the decision to treat differ from other populations? This chapter reviews the prevalence, diagnosis, association with adverse events, and treatment options for anemia in individuals living in long-term care settings.

PREVALENCE IN LONG-TERM CARE SETTING

People older than 65 years are projected to double in number from 46 million in 2014 to 98 million in 2060, or to roughly 1 out of 4 people, whereas those older than 85 years

Disclosure Statement: The authors have nothing to disclose.
[a] Division of Geriatrics and Palliative Care, Department of Medicine, Rhode Island Hospital, The Warren Alpert Medical School of Brown University, POB 438, 593, Eddy Street, Providence, RI 02903, USA; [b] Department of Health Services Policy and Practice, School of Public Health, Providence Veterans Administration Medical Center, Brown University, 6th Floor, Rm 627,121 South Main Street, Providence, RI 02903, USA
* Corresponding author. Division of Geriatrics and Palliative Care, Rhode Island Hospital, POB 438, 593, Eddy Street, Providence, RI 02903.
E-mail address: ananda@lifespan.org

Clin Geriatr Med 35 (2019) 381–389
https://doi.org/10.1016/j.cger.2019.03.008
0749-0690/19/© 2019 Elsevier Inc. All rights reserved.

geriatric.theclinics.com

are projected to triple from 6 million to 20 million.[1] The number of individuals requiring long-term care services numbered 12 million in 2015 and 63% are older than 65 years of age. That number is also expected to increase to 27 million by 2050.[2–4]

Because the population requiring long-term care has multiple morbidities, the prevalence of anemia is expected to be much higher. A systematic review of anemia in older people found prevalence of anemia is highest among nursing home residents with weighted mean of 47%, compared with 12% in community dwellers.[5] The prevalence in another study of 900 nursing home residents reported anemia in 48%.[5,6] Robinson and colleagues[7] examined records of more than 6000 nursing home residents and found 60% with anemia and 43% with chronic kidney disease; more residents with chronic kidney disease had anemia (65%) than those who did not have chronic kidney disease. In 2014, the Centers for Disease Control and Prevention reported that long-term service users totaled 9 million, out of which around 1.4 million people reside in some 15,000 nursing homes in the United States and about two-thirds of these live there permanently.[8]

The high prevalence and nonspecific symptoms of anemia can be attributable to a plethora of other conditions common in nursing home residents; when such symptoms are attributed to other conditions, anemia may not be considered etiologically high enough in the differential diagnosis and accordingly may go undiagnosed. The notion that anemia is an inevitable consequence of aging can be refuted by data that show that most older people have a normal hemoglobin and hematocrit and those who meet the criteria for anemia (Hgb <12 g per dL) have an identifiable cause in most of the cases.[9] It is also not entirely clear what the clinical significance of anemia is in older people when the cause is not found.

ASSOCIATION WITH CHRONIC DISEASE, DELIRIUM, DEMENTIA, AND DECREASED QUALITY OF LIFE

In older adults, anemia has been associated with worsening delirium, dementia, and a declining quality of life. Investigators have suggested anemia is associated with worse outcomes in people with specific comorbid conditions such as heart failure. A study involving heart failure patients showed that anemia was present in 17% of patients, the most of whom (58%) were found to have anemia of chronic disease.[10] The 5-year mortality rate in this large cohort of people with heart failure is 10% higher in those with anemia.[10]

A prospective study of 190 elderly subjects aged older than 70 years with an anemia prevalence of 50% found anemia to be an independent risk factor for delirium. Even after adjusting for age, sex, and diagnosis of dementia, the odds ratio for delirium was found to be significantly associated with anemia.[11] Another study found the degree of anemia correlated with the severity of delirium and length of stay in intensive care unit.[12]

Presence of anemia is also associated with new dementia onset and accelerated cognitive decline.[13,14] A 3-year prospective study involving more than 1400 subjects with normal baseline cognitive function found that those with anemia were twice as likely to develop dementia even after adjusting for age, gender, educational level, comorbid conditions, and nutritional status.[15]

ASSOCIATION WITH FALLS, DECLINE IN PHYSICAL PERFORMANCE, HAZARDS OF HOSPITALIZATIONS, AND INCREASE IN MORTALITY

Several studies linked lower hemoglobin levels to the occurrence of those who fall while hospitalized. Dharmarajan and colleagues[16] compared the risk of falls in hospitalized elderly patients both from the community and from the nursing homes who met WHO defined criteria for anemia. They found that more than half of the patients had a fall during hospital stay and those who experienced a fall had a higher prevalence of anemia (56% vs 38%, P = .001). It also revealed a 1.9-fold increased likelihood of falls in those with anemia and a risk independent of age, race, or place of residence, such as the nursing home.[16]

Studies also indicate an association between anemia and functional decline.[17,18] A prospective study following 1146 patients over a period of 4 years found a significant association between anemia and functional decline even after adjusting for anemia-associated laboratory abnormalities (serum iron, albumin, and lipid) and diseases (malignancy, renal insufficiency, and infectious disease).[18]

Dhamarajan[19] also compared the number of hospitalizations with the severity of anemia in older nursing home and community elderly. The author reported that 60% of nonanemic individuals were hospitalized during the prior 18 months compared with 80% of anemic individuals. Men, African American race, and chronicity of anemia were linked with higher likelihood of hospitalization.[19] It is not clear whether the anemia itself contributes to the hospitalization risk, or the underlying cause of anemia, or both serve as drivers of that risk.

Several studies have shown an association between anemia and increased mortality.[20,21] A study examining the association between hemoglobin and all-cause mortality in 17,000 older adults found increased mortality risk associated with both extremes of hemoglobin.[22]

In each of these outcomes that associates with anemia, there remains work to be done to determine how anemia figures into the risk in terms of causality or as a proxy for some other problem that directly confers risk. In addition, this work does not answer the question of whether treating the anemia or its cause modifies the risk for these outcomes in general, or specifically in the nursing home setting.

CLINICAL PRESENTATION

Anemia is most commonly found incidentally on abnormal screening tests rather than in the evaluation of signs and symptoms associated with acute blood loss or hemolysis.[23] Slowly progressive or chronic anemia is typically less symptomatic, especially in a sedentary nursing home patient, and gradual compensatory mechanisms can allow it to remain clinically silent. Thus, signs and symptoms may not appear until the hemoglobin drops to where the body's mechanisms (increase in blood volume and cardiac output) for homeostasis can no longer adequately compensate. With acute blood loss anemia, laboratory values can lag until after postural hypotension, tachycardia, and dyspnea become evident.[23]

Acute blood loss, such as from a gastrointestinal bleed, can produce an acute, overtly symptomatic presentation. However, most anemic older patients present with milder, more easily missed symptoms such as fatigue, lethargy, weakness, or shortness of breath, which might be easily ascribed to old age.[9] Symptoms of anemia may be inconspicuous in elderly due to reduction in mobility and physical activity secondary to joint pain, muscle atrophy, and other medical conditions and social expectations, such as for those living in the nursing home setting. Furthermore, many institutionalized elderly have cognitive impairment or frank dementia and may not reliably be able to report symptoms or their chronology. Because the symptoms may be attributed to other comorbid conditions such as heart failure, anemia can go unnoticed without a sufficiently detailed history and physical examination and laboratory evaluation.

Anemia evaluation should seek to assess nutritional history, often best acquired from nursing home staff, who also can provide a longitudinal weight record. The nursing home social worker may also know of any alcohol or illicit drug use. The resident or their family may know of a family history of anemia. Certain inherited disorders are common in certain geographic areas and ethnic backgrounds such as thalassemia and G6PD deficiency. Review of systems and physical examination should include blood in the stool or urine, bleeding from gums or mucosal surfaces, splenomegaly, lymphadenopathy, or other signs of infection.[23]

Common red flags that can preclude the onset of symptoms of anemia and prevent an adverse event include a thorough review of comorbid diseases and recent events including hospitalization, procedures, or new medications. Common comorbid diseases that can predispose to anemia are listed in **Table 1**.

Several medications are implicated with anemia (listed in **Table 2**), and therefore, a thorough and regular review of medication should be conducted on every medical encounter and especially after a recent hospitalization.

Common physical signs in the diagnosis of anemia useful in any race because of independence from skin pigmentation include pallor of the conjunctiva, hands, and nailbed.[24] Conjunctival pallor had a likelihood ratio of 4.49 for anemia. Thus, conjunctival pallor is independently sufficient to suspect anemia and trigger a hemoglobin measurement to rule out severe anemia.[25] Other physical examination findings can include strong peripheral pulses, strong and forceful heartbeat, and rarely a compensatory high-output heart failure from tissue hypoxia.[24] Note that severe atherosclerosis, as can be found in older nursing home residents, may attenuate peripheral pulses.

EVALUATION OF ANEMIA

A detailed history and physical examination are followed by laboratory testing with a complete blood count including peripheral blood smear. The results of the initial blood work can further refine the differential diagnosis and may point toward a certain cause or need for further testing. According to NHANES III data collected between 1991 and 1994 and related to the cause of anemia in persons older than 65 years old, the causes of anemia can be roughly classified into 3 categories. Nutritional deficiency occurs in one-third of those with anemia (iron, folate, and vitamin B12), of which half are attributable to iron deficiency anemia. Chronic inflammation (20%) or chronic renal failure (8%) makes up another third of elderly with anemia. The remaining one-third of anemic elderly has an undetermined cause.[26]

The proportion of those with anemia of unknown cause increases with age, and the average age of nursing home residents in the United States is 80 years and older.[26–30] A study involving nursing home residents found that in 45% of those with anemia, the workup of anemia did not yield any identifiable cause.[5]

Table 1	
Common medical diagnoses associated with anemia	
Types of Anemia	**Medical Predispositions**
Microcytic anemia	Low dietary intake of iron Recent blood loss (surgical or trauma) Acute or chronic gastrointestinal bleeding
Macrocytic anemia	Low dietary intake of vitamin B12 or folate
Anemia of chronic disease	Chronic inflammation, cancer, chronic kidney disease
Endocrine disorders	Diabetes mellitus, thyroid disease

Table 2	
Common medications that contribute to anemia	
Drugs associated with gastrointestinal bleeding	Anticoagulants (eg, Coumadin, heparin, novel oral anticoagulants)
	Antiplatelets (eg, aspirin, clopidogrel, abciximab)
	Corticosteroids (eg, hydrocortisone)
	Bisphosphonates (eg, alendronate)
	Nonsteroidal antiinflammatory drugs (eg, ibuprofen)
Drugs that affect folate levels and utilization	Alcohol, phenytoin
Drugs that interfere with folate metabolism	Methotrexate, pentamidine, triamterene, lamotrigine, trimethoprim-sulfamethoxazole, primidone
Drugs that affect folate utilization & metabolism	Phenobarbital, sulfasalazine
Drugs that decrease vitamin B12 absorption	Metformin, colchicine, proton pump inhibitor, histamine blockers
Drugs associated with myelosuppression	Azathioprine, 6-mercaptopurine, cyclophosphamide, busulfan, doxorubicin, zidovudine, methotrexate, hydroxyurea, thioguanine
Alternate therapies linked with anemia	Ginkgo (bleeding), yohimbe (renal failure), black cohosh, and green tea

Data from Saffel D. Putting it into practice: strategizing a successful anemia management protocol in the long-term care setting. Consult Pharm 2008;23 Suppl A:18–23.

The evaluation of nursing home residents should consider factors not typically germane for younger and healthier patients. Before ordering a barrage of tests, consider whether the test and treatment for the diagnosis the patient is being tested for is warranted and would be tolerated by the patient. For example, would it make sense to do a bone marrow transplant in an elderly patient with advanced dementia? If the patient is bed-bound would the patient achieve meaningful clinical or quality of life gains with an improvement in their hemoglobin concentration? In some cases it may be prudent to test for a cause by evaluating a response to empirical treatment such as giving iron replacement therapy and monitoring hemoglobin and reticulocyte count for a few months. In such cases it would be appropriate to set a target response, which determines failure (stop treatment) or success (diagnosis is made; continue or stop treatment). It is important to weigh the risks and benefits of testing and treatment in due consideration of patient's expected longevity and whether doing more would add meaningful quality of life. Therefore, as in the management of any other serious illness, evaluation of anemia should be done considering expected quality of life and feeling of well-being and patient's goals of care (**Fig. 1**). If patient is unable to participate, then the patient's family and/or health care proxy should use substituted judgment in deciding management in accordance with patient's values.

Lastly, cost of care should be aligned with benefit to the patient. It is often difficult to choose which way to proceed. For example, should one consider long-term transfusions for an elderly nursing home patient if the tests indicated a myelodysplastic syndrome that is otherwise unresponsive to other interventions?

As discussed earlier, anemia is associated with many adverse outcomes in long-term care residents, so further testing for a treatable cause may be warranted.

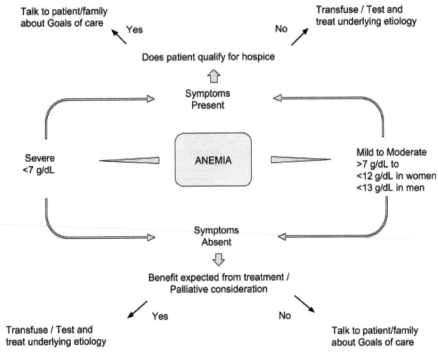

Fig. 1. Evaluating anemia in the long-term care setting.

However, the authors of this chapter have divergent opinions on where to draw the line on both formal anemia evaluation and treatment. Which tests to order to evaluate anemia is dealt with in detail elsewhere in this book.

TREATMENT

Treatment decisions will take into account the subjective considerations of patient wishes, goals of care, and whether it will improve the quality of life. Treatment of anemia found on routine laboratory testing of apparently asymptomatic long-term care residents should be tailored and different clinicians may not be equally aggressive. Aside from acute blood loss such as from a gastrointestinal bleed or following a large bone fracture, when present, signs and symptoms from more insidious causes of anemia that may also suggest anemia are typically nonspecific. When this is the case, a low blood count may be coincident with a decline in cognitive status or change in activities of daily living, intentional or unintentional dietary changes, new onset or an increase in falls, or frequent infections, so who should be evaluated depends on clinical suspicion and anticipated benefit from intervention.[31] So when these symptoms are due to anemia, they should factor into the decision on whether to treat the anemia.

Specific treatment of anemia depends on the cause. Anemia due to acute blood loss may require volume resuscitation or blood transfusions. Iron deficiency anemia responds well to ferrous sulfate, 325 mg, once daily and increase in daily intake of iron-rich foods (meat, fish, spinach, kale, beans, or iron-fortified cereal). It is recommended to take iron supplements 2 hours after calcium supplements and is better absorbed if taken together with vitamin C. A common side effect of iron therapy is constipation, which should be monitored and treated appropriately. Patients should be made aware that supplemental iron can make the stool appear dark, so they may not get alarmed and concerned that they may be bleeding per rectum. Conversely, iron supplement can mask upper gastrointestinal bleed, so hemoglobin should be monitored routinely.

Animal protein is the main source of vitamin B12, hence, vegetarians or vegans and elderly who do not consume enough protein can be or become deficient. Vitamin B12 deficiency can be treated with high doses of cyanocobalamin orally (as is common in Europe) or with intramuscular administration of 1000 mg/mL of vitamin B12. It is also available as deep subcutaneous injection and can be given weekly until normal and then once a month.[31] Folate deficiency can be easily treated with 1 mg of folate daily and levels can be rechecked in 2 to 3 weeks. Dietary folate levels can be replenished by eating green leafy vegetables, whole grains, and nuts. Nutritional management of anemias is more straightforward in the long-term care setting as diet and weight are monitored and can be tracked over time, so there is greater certainty about the adherence to specific interventions than in the outpatient settings.

Anemia associated with chronic kidney disease may require erythropoiesis-stimulating agents (ESA); however, such agents are typically expensive and should be used judiciously and reserved for patients who are expected to have a meaningful benefit in quality of life and physical function from the treatment. Iron deficiency should be excluded by serum ferritin of greater than 100 μg/L and total saturation of greater than 20%, before starting ESA, and the dose of ESA should be titrated to hemoglobin levels between 11 and 12 g/dL.[32] These agents are costly and come with a "black box" warning on the label for recommended treatment targets and safety risks by Food and Drug Administration. When anemia is caused by other chronic diseases, the appropriate way will be to treat the underlying condition, if possible. Overall, the treatment should be based on evaluation of individual patient as well as the discussion between the clinician, patient, and/or family.

SUMMARY

Anemia is prevalent among the elderly; however, the signs and symptoms of anemia are often nonspecific and especially in frail elderly such as those living in nursing homes may be attributed to physical decline associated with increasing age. Anemia is often underdiagnosed. As it can be an insidious sign of an underlying disorder with a discernible cause, it may be easily remedied and may warrant formal workup. Anemia is a disease and although the symptoms may be clandestine due to multimorbidity among the elderly, undiagnosed anemia has tangible and perceptible consequences including poor quality of life and early death. Because of the high prevalence of concomitant chronic diseases, the detection of anemia in the elderly poses a diagnostic challenge. A viable approach in diagnosing and treating anemia includes a consideration of the diagnostic burden and potential benefit to the overall functioning and quality of life of the patient.

REFERENCES

1. Mather M, Jacobsen LA, Ard KMP. Population Bulletin 2015;23. Available at: https://www.prb.org/unitedstates-population-bulletin/. Accessed April 28, 2019.
2. David S, Sheikh F, Mahajan D, et al. Whom do we serve? Describing the target population for post-acute and long-term care, focusing on nursing facility settings, in the era of population health in the United States. J Am Med Dir Assoc 2016;17(7):574–80.

3. Hollowell JG, van Assendelft OW, Gunter EW, et al. Hematological and iron-related analytes–reference data for persons aged 1 year and over: United States, 1988-94. Vital Health Stat 11 2005;(247):1–156.
4. Salive ME. Anemia and hemoglobin levels in older persons: relationship with age, gender, and health status. J Am Geriatr Soc 1992. https://doi.org/10.1111/j.1532-5415.1992.tb02017.x.
5. Artz AS, Fergusson D, Drinka PJ, et al. Mechanisms of unexplained anemia in the nursing home: anemia in nursing home residents. J Am Geriatr Soc 2004;52(3): 423–7.
6. Kalchthaler T, Tan ME. Anemia in institutionalized elderly patients. J Am Geriatr Soc 1980;28(3):108–13.
7. Robinson B, Artz AS, Culleton B, et al. Prevalence of anemia in the nursing home: contribution of chronic kidney disease: prevalence of CKD and anemia in SNFS. J Am Geriatr Soc 2007;55(10):1566–70.
8. Harris-Kojetin LD, Sengupta M, Park-Lee E, National Center for Health Statistics (U.S.). Long-term care providers and services users in the United States: data from the national study of long-term care providers, 2013-2014. Vital Health Stat 3 2016;(38). x-xii, 1-105.
9. Smith DL. Anemia in the elderly. Am Fam Physician 2000;62(7):1565–72.
10. Ezekowitz JA, McAlister FA, Armstrong PW. Anemia is common in heart failure and is associated with poor outcomes: insights from a cohort of 12 065 patients with new-onset heart failure. Circulation 2003;107(2):223–5.
11. Joosten E, Lemiengre J, Nelis T, et al. Is anaemia a risk factor for delirium in an acute geriatric population? Gerontology 2006;52(6):382–5.
12. Granberg Axèll AIR, Malmros CW, Bergbom IL, et al. Intensive care unit syndrome/delirium is associated with anemia, drug therapy and duration of ventilation treatment. Acta Anaesthesiol Scand 2002;46(6):726–31.
13. Hong CH, Falvey C, Harris TB, et al. Anemia and risk of dementia in older adults: findings from the Health ABC study. Neurology 2013;81(6):528–33.
14. Shah RC, Buchman AS, Wilson RS, et al. Hemoglobin level in older persons and incident Alzheimer disease: prospective cohort analysis. Neurology 2011;77(3): 219–26.
15. Atti A, Palmer K, Volpato S, et al. Anaemia increases the risk of dementia in cognitively intact elderly. Neurobiol Aging 2006;27(2):278–84.
16. Dharmarajan TS, Avula S, Norkus EP. Anemia increases risk for falls in hospitalized older adults: an evaluation of falls in 362 hospitalized, ambulatory, long-term care, and community patients. J Am Med Dir Assoc 2006;7(5):287–93.
17. Thein M, Ershler WB, Artz AS, et al. Diminished quality of life and physical function in community-dwelling elderly with anemia. Medicine 2009;88(2):107–14.
18. Penninx BWJH, Guralnik JM, Onder G, et al. Anemia and decline in physical performance among older persons. Am J Med 2003;115(2):104–10.
19. Dharmarajan TS. Anemia in the long-term care setting: routine screening and differential diagnosis. Consult Pharm 2008;23(Suppl A):5–10.
20. Riva E, Tettamanti M, Mosconi P, et al. Association of mild anemia with hospitalization and mortality in the elderly: the Health and Anemia population-based study. Haematologica 2009;94(1):22–8.
21. Denny SD, Kuchibhatla MN, Cohen HJ. Impact of anemia on mortality, cognition, and function in community-dwelling elderly. Am J Med 2006;119(4):327–34.
22. Culleton BF. Impact of anemia on hospitalization and mortality in older adults. Blood 2006;107(10):3841–6.

23. Adamson JW, Longo DL. Anemia and polycythemia. In: Jameson J, Fauci AS, Kasper DL, et al, editors. Harrison's principles of internal medicine, 20e. New York: McGraw-Hill. Available at: http://accessmedicine.mhmedical.com/content.aspx?bookid=2129&sectionid=192014145. Accessed April 28, 2019.

24. Strobach RS. The value of the physical examination in the diagnosis of anemia. Correlation of the physical findings and the hemoglobin concentration. Arch Intern Med 1988;148(4):831–2.

25. Sheth TN, Choudhry NK, Bowes M, et al. The relation of conjunctival pallor to the presence of anemia. J Gen Intern Med 1997;12(2):102–6.

26. Guralnik JM. Prevalence of anemia in persons 65 years and older in the United States: evidence for a high rate of unexplained anemia. Blood 2004;104(8): 2263–8.

27. Ganz T. The role of hepcidin in iron sequestration during infections and in the pathogenesis of anemia of chronic disease. Isr Med Assoc J 2002;4(11):1043–5.

28. Chua E, Clague JE, Sharma AK, et al. Serum transferrin receptor assay in iron deficiency anaemia and anaemia of chronic disease in the elderly. QJM 1999; 92(10):587–94.

29. Hanif E, Ayyub M, Anwar M, et al. Evaluation of serum transferrin receptor concentration in diagnosing and differentiating iron deficiency anaemia from anaemia of chronic disorders. J Pak Med Assoc 2005;55(1):13–6.

30. Rockey DC, Cello JP. Evaluation of the gastrointestinal tract in patients with iron-deficiency anemia. N Engl J Med 1993;329(23):1691–5.

31. Saffel D. Putting it into practice: strategizing a successful anemia management protocol in the long-term care setting. Consult Pharm 2008;23(Suppl A):18–23.

32. Mikhail, Brown C, Williams JA, et al. Clinical practice guideline: anemia of chronic kidney disease 2017. Available at: https://renal.org/wp-content/uploads/2017/06/anaemia-of-chronic-kidney-disease5d84a231181561659443ff000014d4d8.pdf. Accessed December 14, 2018.

Implications of Anemia in the Elderly Undergoing Surgery

Yilin Eileen Sim, MMed (Anaesthesiology), Hairil Rizal Abdullah, MMed (Anaesthesiology)*

KEYWORDS

- Preoperative anemia • Iron deficiency • Elderly • Intravenous iron • Erythropoietin
- Anemia clinic • Patient blood management

KEY POINTS

- Preoperative anemia is common in the elderly, and iron deficiency or concomitant iron deficiency with anemia of chronic disease are frequent causes.
- Patients should be screened for the anemia early, ideally as soon as they are listed for surgery, and the cause of preoperative anemia can be identified with additional iron indices, such as serum iron, transferrin, ferritin, transferrin saturation, serum folate, and vitamin B_{12} levels. Major, nonurgent surgery should be postponed to allow the diagnosis and treatment of anemia and iron deficiency.
- Oral iron is the first-line treatment of preoperative iron-deficiency anemia. However, in patients who have limited time to surgery, are unable to tolerate the side effects of oral iron, or who have no response to oral iron replacement, intravenous (IV) iron is considered.
- IV iron is efficacious and safe and is given to patients preoperatively or postoperatively. It is associated with significant hemoglobin improvement after discharge, compared with no supplement.

PREVALENCE OF ANEMIA IN THE SURGICAL SETTING

Anemia is fairly common in the surgical population.[1] Among elderly patients older than 70 years, this prevalence could be 47%. Unlike in the younger, reproductive age groups where anemia is more prevalent in the female population, in the elderly older than 50 years, the frequency of anemia between men and women is almost identical, and may even be higher in males compared with females in the very elderly patients more than 70 years old (**Fig. 1**).[1] The incidence of anemia is also particularly common in surgeries that are more frequently performed in the older age group, such as resection of colorectal cancers and hip and knee arthroplasty.[2–5]

Disclosure Statement: The authors have no commercial or financial conflicts of interest and any funding sources.
Department of Anaesthesiology, Singapore General Hospital, Outram Road, Singapore 169608, Singapore
* Corresponding author.
E-mail address: hairil.rizal.abdullah@singhealth.com.sg

geriatric.theclinics.com

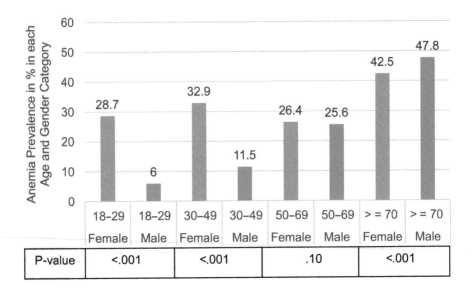

Fig. 1. Prevalence of anemia according to age and gender groups in an Asian population. (*From* Sim YE, Wee HE, Ang AL, et al. Prevalence of preoperative anemia, abnormal mean corpuscular volume and red cell distribution width among surgical patients in Singapore, and their influence on one year mortality. PLoS One 2017;12(8):e0182543; with permission.)

DEFINITIONS OF ANEMIA

In the general population, anemia is defined by the World Health Organization as a hemoglobin (Hb) concentration of less than 13 g/dL for men, less than 12 g/dL for nonpregnant women, and less than 11 g/dL for pregnant women.[6] These definitions are widely used in epidemiologic studies. However, as a threshold for preoperative diagnosis and treatment, this may not be suitable for women undergoing surgical procedures in which moderate-to-high blood loss is expected. Women have lower circulating blood volumes than men, but the same procedures performed in either sex often result in comparable amounts of blood loss.[7] Therefore, when measured as a proportion of circulating blood volume, blood losses are proportionally higher in women and may result in higher perioperative blood transfusion rates.[8,9] This has led to calls in recent international guidelines for a nongender-based approach, with a single cutoff of less than 13 g/dL when diagnosing anemia in the preoperative population.[10]

CAUSES OF ANEMIA

About one-third of anemia in the elderly is ascribed to nutritional deficiency (iron, folate, B_{12}), another one-third to chronic disease (inflammatory states, renal failure resulting in reduced erythropoietin production) and hemoglobinopathies, and the last third remains unexplained.[11,12] Of these, iron deficiency anemia is the most common in the surgical population presenting for major elective surgery.[3,13] Absolute iron deficiency, defined as the lack of storage iron, is common in the elderly because of a combination of malnutrition; malabsorption; or chronic gastrointestinal blood losses secondary to antiplatelet, anticoagulation, or neoplastic lesions.[11,14] However, "functional" or "relative" iron deficiency is defined as the occurrence of iron-restricted erythropoiesis in the presence of normal or even increased amounts of body iron stores.[14,15] This could be caused by iron sequestration in the reticuloendothelial system, where there is a block of iron release from macrophages and hepatocytes, typically during chronic inflammation, or by increased/ineffective/stimulated erythropoiesis, with iron demand exceeding the supply (ie, during hemoglobinopathies, chronic hemolytic anemias, or treatment with erythropoiesis stimulating agents [ESAs]). Iron sequestration is thought to be partially mediated by a small peptide hormone secreted by hepatocytes called hepcidin. Hepcidin increases the endocytosis and degradation of ferroportin, the membrane protein responsible for absorption of oral iron in duodenal enterocytes and release of iron from macrophages and hepatocytes.[16,17] Production of hepcidin is strongly stimulated by proinflammatory states.[14,18]

SIGNIFICANCE OF PREOPERATIVE ANEMIA

Preoperative anemia is associated with excess risks for mortality in cardiac and noncardiac surgery.[1,19–24] The pooled odds ratio of 30-day mortality for preoperative anemia is 2.20 (95% confidence interval, 1.68–2.88) on a recent meta-analysis.[25] Among elderly patients undergoing noncardiac surgery, as hematocrit levels decrease to less than 39% or greater than 51%, the incidence of 30-day mortality and cardiac event rates increase linearly, alluding to a J-shaped relationship between anemia and mortality.[2] Similar J-shaped relationship between anemia and mortality has also been found in elderly patients in the community setting.[26] Preoperative anemia has also been associated with postoperative complications, such as acute myocardial infarction, acute ischemic stroke, acute kidney injury, postoperative admission to intensive care, and prolonged length of hospital stay, although the effect size for these events is smaller.[4,25,27] Moreover, it also associated with reduced quality of life, fatigue, depression, decreased muscle strength, self-reported disability, and decline of physical performance in community and hospitalized elderly patients.[5,28,29]

Most importantly, preoperative anemia is the strongest predictor of perioperative blood transfusion.[4,7,30] A large meta-analysis involving 949,000 patients and 24 studies found that the odds of receiving blood transfusion in patients anemic preoperatively is 5.04 (4.12–6.17; I[2] = 96%; $P < .001$).[23] Transfusion is associated with increased mortality risks for those with preoperative hematocrit levels between 30% and 35.9% and 500 mL of blood loss.[31]

Furthermore, elderly patients undergoing surgery are particularly vulnerable to blood loss and anemia's adverse effects, because they have limited physiologic reserve, and a higher prevalence of underlying coronary disease.[32] Hence, patient blood management (PBM) programs to diagnose and manage preoperative anemia are especially relevant in this population.

BEST PRACTICES ON PREOPERATIVE ANEMIA MANAGEMENT

Preoperative anemia is best managed as part of a comprehensive PBM program within an institution.[25] PBM is an evidence-based, individualized approach to minimize a patient's exposure to blood products by focusing on the three pillars of PBM. The three pillars are: maximizing total red cell mass, minimizing perioperative blood loss, and improving tolerance of anemia.[33] Consensus guidelines in PBM have been updated recently to emphasize effective treatment of preoperative anemia, which requires advanced screening, diagnosis, and initiation of therapy weeks before elective surgery. Several institutions have established preoperative anemia clinics to manage this problem, such as the Preoperative Anemia clinic in Duke University Hospital,[34] Preoperative Anemia Management Clinic at the University of Iowa Hospitals & Clinics,[35] and University Hospital Frankfurt.[36] These clinics have in common a preoperative patient pathway that has a protocol-guided screening process, diagnostic algorithms, referral pathway, and treatment. A recent meta-analysis demonstrated reduction in the transfusion need of red blood cells (RBC) and lower perioperative complications and mortality rate among patients who underwent a comprehensive PBM program.[37]

SCREENING FOR ANEMIA ETIOLOGY

Patients who are planned for surgery with a significant risk of bleeding should be screened for preoperative anemia as early as possible. Ideally, screening and treatment of anemia should begin even while patients are considering the surgery, although this is rarely practiced.

When anemia is detected on a full blood count screen preoperatively, additional investigations should be ordered to determine the cause. Serum ferritin and transferrin saturation (TSat) are commonly used for an initial evaluation of iron status. Serum ferritin less than 30 μg/L is the most sensitive and specific test used for the identification of absolute iron deficiency and if present, no further laboratory work-up is needed.[38] However, ferritin is an acute-phase reactant and may frequently be raised in settings of inflammation. Thus, when serum ferritin levels are greater than 30 μg/L, its value should be corroborated with other iron indices, such as TSat. TSat less than 20% may indicate insufficient iron supply to support normal erythropoiesis. Hence, in the presence of inflammation (C-reactive protein >5 mg/L) and/or TSat less than 20%, a serum ferritin level less than 100 μg/L may still be indicative of concomitant iron deficiency and anemia of chronic inflammation. However, ferritin levels greater than 100 μg/L, even in the presence of TSat less than 20%, is more likely to be associated with anemia of chronic inflammation or functional iron deficiency, which may occur during treatment with ESAs, or in patients with end-stage renal disease on hemodialysis.[10,39] Other investigations that can be done simultaneously are serum B_{12} and folate levels to rule out anemia of malnutrition.

When the interpretation of iron studies is uncertain because of recent blood transfusion that may affect iron studies transiently,[40] or in the presence of chronic inflammation, malignancy, or chronic kidney disease, additional tests may be helpful, although these may not routinely be available in the hospital laboratory. These tests include measuring the percentage of hypochromic red cells (HRC) and reticulocyte Hb (CHr) content with flow cytometry; assessing serum hepcidin; levels of soluble transferrin receptor (sTfR); and calculating the ratio of serum transferrin receptor level to the log of ferritin (sTfR/log Ft), the so-called ferritin index.[10,39,41] The value of these tests is discussed later.

TREATMENT OF IRON-DEFICIENCY ANEMIA

Iron-deficiency anemia may be addressed by giving patients oral or intravenous (IV) iron supplementation. The choice of the route of application should be individualized based on the degree of preoperative anemia, the remaining time before surgery, and the patient's ability to absorb and tolerate oral iron.[10]

For oral iron therapy, a course of 40 to 60 mg elemental iron daily, or 80 to 100 mg elemental iron on alternate days is recommended for 6 to 8 weeks.[10] This is because only 10% of oral iron is absorbed in the body.[42] Given that the estimated iron deficit is about 700 mg in a patient with mild anemia with Hb 11 g/dL, to about 1300 mg in a patient with severe anemia and Hb of 7 g/dL, the time taken for oral iron to replace the iron deficit would be proportionately longer depending on the severity of anemia.[43] In a group of hospitalized octogenarians with iron-deficiency anemia who were given oral iron replacement of between 15 mg/d and 150 mg/d for 2 months, the average rise in Hb was modest, about 1.3 to 1.4 g/dL.[44] This timeline may not be clinically acceptable depending on the surgical indication. Furthermore, adherence to oral iron is suboptimal, with 20% of patients failing to complete the full course because of side effects, such as abdominal pain, constipation, and nausea.[44-46] Side effects are more common at higher doses of oral iron. Oral iron absorption is also reduced when taken together with antacids, proton pump inhibitors, or in the presence of gastrointestinal diseases.[42,47,48] Oral absorption of iron may also be limited in elderly patients with multiple comorbidities because of age-related elevation of hepcidin levels.[41] IV iron is superior in this regard because it has no gastrointestinal side effects and is highly efficacious at replenishing iron stores.[49]

IV iron has become standard front-line therapy for iron-deficiency anemia in inflammatory bowel disease because there is some evidence that oral iron may increase clinical disease activity in inflammatory bowel disease.[50,51] Patients who have undergone either Roux-en-Y or biliopancreatic bariatric surgery are also frequently iron deficient because of the bypass of the duodenum from normal alimentary flow, which is the usual site of oral iron absorption. Frequently, the iron-deficiency anemia in these patient is resistant to oral iron therapy because of malabsorption, and IV iron is recommended.[52] The use of IV iron in patients undergoing hemodialysis may also enhance erythropoiesis, and lower requirements for ESAs.[39,53] In the preoperative setting, because the use of IV iron circumvents the problem of iron absorption, it is more effective in replenishing iron stores and increases Hb levels more quickly than oral iron,[54-56] potentially negating the need for lengthy postponement of surgery.

Older formulations of IV iron, such as the high-molecular-weight iron dextran, were frequently associated with severe infusion reactions. Newer products, such as ferric carboxymaltose and iron isomaltoside, have much lower frequency of adverse reactions, and can deliver larger doses of iron within a single dose, between 750 mg and 1000 mg.[57,58]

Infused IV iron has a circulatory half-life of approximately 2 weeks. During that time, transferrin is regularly supplied with elemental iron for erythropoiesis, and peak ferritin response occurs 7 to 9 days after IV iron.[59,60] Ferric carboxymaltose infusion should not exceed 1000 mg in a single infusion, whereas for iron isomaltoside, each infusion should be limited to 20 mg/kg. Thus, if the patient's estimated total iron deficit (based on popular formulas, such as the Ganzoni formula) exceeds a single dose limit, a second infusion is scheduled 1 to 2 weeks after the first.[57]

Oral iron therapy should be supervised for compliance and effectiveness because of the high incidence of gastrointestinal side effects.[42] If side effects are significant enough to limit compliance, the physician can change the formulation of oral iron to enteric-coated, encourage consumption with food, reduce the dosage, or reduce the frequency of dosing to every other day.[61] If there is sufficient time before surgery, a repeat full blood count 2 to 3 weeks after initiation of therapy to monitor Hb response is considered. Therapeutic doses of iron should increase Hb levels by 0.7 to 1.0 g/dL per week. Reticulocytosis occurs within 7 to 10 days after initiation of iron therapy.[62] If the response is poor, causes for failure, such as noncompliance, malabsorption, ongoing blood loss, and dual-pathology impeding bone marrow response, should be elicited, and alternative treatment, such as IV iron, may be considered.[61]

STIMULATION OF ERYTHROPOIESIS

ESAs may be considered for patients with anemia with iron sequestration secondary to anemia of chronic disease.[10] The latest consensus statement gave a conditional recommendation for the use of short-acting erythropoietin plus iron supplementation in adult preoperative elective major orthopedic patients with preoperative Hb levels less than 13 g/dL only.[25] A systematic review of randomized controlled trials (RCTs) involving the use of erythropoietin in patients scheduled for total hip or knee arthroplasty found that preoperative use of erythropoietin was associated with lower exposure to allogeneic blood transfusion (odds ratio, 0.41) and higher Hb concentration after surgery (standardized mean difference, 0.86; $P < .001$).[63] However, ESA therapy may be associated with a small increased risk of deep vein thrombosis or pulmonary embolism in patients with cancer (pooled relative risk for a thromboembolic event with ESA use was 1.51),[64] but not in patients undergoing elective orthopedic surgery or colorectal cancer surgery.[63,65] Several RCTs have also demonstrated that patients with cancer-related anemia have reduced overall survival when receiving ESA treatment.[66–69] Hence, most guidelines remain cautious recommending erythropoietin use in patients with history of thrombosis or cancer-related anemia.[10]

CURRENT CHALLENGES IN IMPLEMENTING THESE BEST PRACTICES

Although most international guidelines suggest early detection and correction of anemia before surgery, this practice has not been uniformly adopted worldwide.[10,25,70,71] One of the chief obstacles to preoperative optimization of anemia is the amount of time available between presentation and surgery. For patients who require emergency surgeries, the time between presentation and surgery may be only a matter of mere hours. For elective surgery, the time from diagnosis to surgery varies depending on the indication of the surgery. Surgeries for cancer are time-sensitive, and cannot be delayed too long for optimization of anemia. Because the average time for Hb levels to rise by 1 g with IV iron therapy is 2 to 4 weeks, unless IV iron therapy is given sufficiently in advance of surgery, Hb levels may not rise adequately to reduce the need for intraoperative transfusion. This is supported by reports from preoperative anemia clinics. One such clinic from the University Hospital Frankfurt found that patients who received IV iron within 2 weeks of surgery had a mean rise in Hb of 0.2 (interquartile range, 0.3–0.7) g/dL, whereas patients who received IV iron greater than 14 days from surgery had a mean Hb rise of 1.3 (interquartile range, 0.4–2.8) g/dL. However, they were unable to demonstrate a statistically significant reduction in RBC transfusion intraoperatively and postoperatively.[36]

Not all studies that systematically treated preoperative anemia with oral or IV iron found a reduction in perioperative blood transfusion. As summarized in a recent meta-analysis published in 2018 that examined the effect of preoperative treatment of anemia with iron formulations in six RCTs and one observational trial, only two trials found a reduction in RBC transfusions and one trial reported a reduction in a subgroup analysis.[72] Of the RCTs that reported a positive effect on transfusion, one was conducted in patients undergoing abdominal surgery, who were randomized to receiving either IV iron or standard care. The trial was terminated early because of significantly better outcomes in the IV iron arm. The study found a 60% reduction in allogenic blood transfusion in the IV iron group compared with the usual care group (31.25% vs 12.5%), through an improvement in Hb of 0.8 g/dL with IV iron compared with 0.1 g/dL with usual care ($P = .01$) by the day of admission.[73] The other RCT that found a significant reduction in RBC was in total knee arthroplasty, and the intervention was IV iron and erythropoietin compared with no treatment.[74]

The impact on RBC transfusion was nonsignificant in similarly well-conducted contemporaneous RCTs, including one by Bernabeu-Wittel and colleagues[75] on elderly patients older than 65 years with hip fracture, randomized to either IV iron and erythropoietin, IV iron alone, or placebo. Two RCTs involving patients undergoing colorectal cancer surgery also found no difference in RBC transfusion between patients randomized to IV iron and none, or between IV iron and oral iron.[76,77] In both RCTs, the average time between therapy and surgery was 2 to 3 weeks. In the study by Keelers and coworkers,[76] with a median study duration of 21 days in both oral and IV iron groups, the median treatment rise in Hb for IV iron (1.55 [interquartile range, 0.93–2.58] g/dL) was significantly higher compared with oral administration (0.50 [-0.13 to 1.33] g/dL; $P<.001$). Nevertheless, Froessler and colleagues[73] and Bernabeau-Wittel and colleagues[75] demonstrate that after surgery, patients who received preoperative IV iron supplementation have better Hb levels than patients that did not on discharge, and up to 2 months after surgery.

In light of the lasting impact of IV iron on postoperative Hb recovery, patients who undergo emergency surgery may still stand to benefit from postoperative treatment of their iron deficiency. A trial by Khalafallah and colleagues that randomized patients who had undergone hip fracture surgery to IV iron or standard care on the first postoperative day found that patients who received IV iron had better Hb levels at 1 month after surgery and reduced postoperative blood transfusion in-hospital.[78] Additionally, in the FAIRY trial, in patients who developed postoperative acute isovolemic anemia after gastrectomy, administration of IV iron postoperatively led to greater improvement in Hb level at 3 months and reduced incidence of alternative anemia management, such as oral iron, transfusion, or both, compared with placebo.[59]

Another major obstacle for the implementation of preoperative anemia pathways is logistical constraints. Ideally, a preoperative anemia clinic should have a comprehensive armamentarium of interventions, including IV iron therapy, erythropoietin injections, gastroenterology and hematology consultations, and a pathway for the delay of elective operation when indicated.[79] Administration of IV iron in the preoperative setting requires logistical planning. A space and setup equipped to deliver IV infusion needs to be created. In addition, clinic nurses must be taught to administer the medication and monitor for side effects afterward. A referral pathway with proper inclusion and exclusion criteria needs to be established. To increase preoperative anemia management opportunities, some centers have automatic electronic medical record alerts when patients are scheduled for elective high blood loss surgeries to remind surgeons to refer to anemia clinics.[35] The physician responsible for overseeing the prescription of oral or IV iron has to be identified, who may be anesthesiologists, hematologists, or perioperative medicine physicians. Finally, when a surgery is purely elective, considerations should be in place to allow for postponement of the surgery for adequate Hb response, which may be after 1 to 2 months. All these can only be achieved if there is multidisciplinary collaboration and support from hospital administrators. Fortunately, there is increasing evidence that preoperative anemia clinics are cost effective, by reducing blood transfusion and hospital length of stay, and may even be sustainable through revenue generation from administration of IV iron and erythropoietin.[34,35]

No management of anemia is complete without evaluation of the underlying cause. When absolute iron-deficiency anemia is present in the elderly, an early referral to a gastroenterologist should be done to rule out gastrointestinal pathologies as a source of chronic blood loss.[80,81] In one cohort of elderly patients with iron-deficiency anemia, 57% had upper gastrointestinal system lesions, 27% colonic lesions, and 15% had gastrointestinal malignancy.[82] If a malignancy is suspected, management of this may take precedence over the original surgery. Patients with existing hematologic or oncologic disease, with severe unexplained anemia (Hb <8.0 g/dL), with evidence of hemolysis, or with decrease in multiple cell lines (neutropenia, thrombocytopenia, RBC aplastic anemia) should be evaluated by a hematologist. Finally, patients with new diagnosis of significant renal impairment (estimated glomerular filtration rate <60 mL/min) should be referred to a nephrologist.[34,71]

KNOWLEDGE GAPS AND FUTURE DIRECTIONS
Identifying Responders to Intravenous Iron Therapy

Because of the increasing number of elderly patients undergoing surgery each year, the burden of preoperative anemia is similarly increasing. Because iron-deficiency anemia has emerged as a potentially modifiable cause of anemia, there is an urgent need to find the most cost-effective test, with the best sensitivity and specificity, to diagnose iron deficiency and identify potential responders to IV iron therapy. This is especially important in the presence of anemia of chronic disease, because traditional markers, such as ferritin and transferrin, are unreliable in chronic inflammation.[10]

Recent studies have suggested the utility of readily available indices in full blood count, such as the RBC distribution width, percentage of HRC, and CHr content. In the setting of microcytic anemia, high red cell distribution width has been shown to have a sensitivity of 94% to predict iron deficiency, and IV iron repletion therapy effectively reduces this index.[83–85] HRC and CHr content are also suitable candidates. The NICE guidelines in the United Kingdom have adopted thresholds of HRC greater than 6% and CHr less than 29 pg to diagnose iron deficiency in chronic kidney disease.[39] These cutoffs has been found to be more cost effective than ferritin level alone at predicting responsiveness to IV iron in patients on hemodialysis.[86] Unfortunately, the lack of analyzer availability and the need for the analysis to be performed within 6 hours after blood sampling preclude their widespread adoption into routine clinical practice. These tests are also unreliable in patients with hemoglobinopathies, such as thalassemia or thalassemia trait.[39]

Newer test candidates for identification of patients who may respond to IV iron include serum hepcidin assays and sTfR. Serum hepcidin is significantly elevated in the elderly with anemia of inflammation, anemia of kidney disease, and in those with unexplained anemia compared with those without anemia.[87] A recent study also found that patients with lower serum hepcidin had better Hb response after IV iron administration.[88] To date, measurement of serum hepcidin levels has not been standardized yet. Use of immunochemical methods may lead to higher levels than mass spectrometry because of inabilities to distinguish hepcidin-25 from its isoforms hepcidin-20 and -22, which are prevalent in chronic kidney disease or chronic inflammation. Hepcidin concentration also demonstrates significant circadian rhythm. Thus, large studies are still needed to establish universal hepcidin reference ranges to enable physicians around the world to compare hepcidin concentrations and to collectively define useful cutoffs for the use of hepcidin in diagnosis of iron disorders.[41] Transferrin receptor (TfR) is the principal means by which various cells acquire iron, especially erythroid precursors in the bone marrow for Hb production. Cell surface TfR concentration is inversely correlated with the iron requirements of the cell. Circulating sTfR level reflects total body TfR concentration, and its level is elevated in various conditions, such as iron-deficient erythropoiesis, or any other causes of increased erythropoiesis. An assay of sTfR may be useful in distinguishing between the anemia of chronic inflammation, iron-deficiency anemia, and when anemia of chronic inflammation and iron-deficiency anemia coexist, because it is normal in the first, and elevated in the latter two. This is because in contrast to serum ferritin and transferrin levels whose levels are altered by presence of inflammation, sTfR levels are not affected by hepcidin or inflammation.[89] STfR levels have been found in preliminary studies to be a predictor of Hb response to IV iron. In a group of patients with stage 3 to 4 chronic kidney disease who were administered IV iron, lower Hepicidin-25 and ferritin levels, and higher sTfR and sTfR/Hepcidin-25 ratio were significant predictors of favorable Hb response within a month after IV iron administration in patients with chronic kidney disease.[90] sTfR is also sensitive to the effect of IV iron, and post-IV iron levels were significantly lower compared with pre-IV iron levels in patients with inflammatory bowel disease.[91]

Finally, there is increasing recognition of the entity of patients with iron-deficiency without anemia.[92] This group may have chronic nonspecific symptoms of weakness, fatigue, difficulty in concentrating, headache, muscle, joint pains, restless leg syndrome, and even poor work productivity because of lower delivery of oxygen to body tissues and decreased activity of iron-containing enzymes.[38,93] The extent to which these nonhematologic effects of iron deficiency are manifested before anemia develops is unclear. The benefit of iron repletion is especially marked in patients with heart failure.[94] The CONFIRM-HF study shows that the treatment of stable, symptomatic, iron-deficient patients with heart failure with IV iron resulted in sustainable improvement in functional capacity over a 1-year period. These favorable results were consistent across patients with and without anemia.[95] This has also been corroborated in the earlier FAIR-HF trial.[96] The prevalence of iron-deficiency without anemia in the elderly is still not known. The cost-effectiveness of a screening strategy to diagnose and treat this condition preoperatively is an area of research that has not been addressed.

SUMMARY

Anemia of the elderly is common and is associated with exposure to blood transfusion and significant perioperative morbidity and mortality risks. These patients would benefit from early diagnosis and workup of the cause of preoperative anemia in a systematic fashion. Increasingly, many centers are establishing preoperative anemia clinics as part of an overall PBM program because iron-deficiency anemia is amenable to treatment with either oral or IV iron. Certain subgroups of patients would benefit from IV iron more, however, further research is needed to guide the identification of this group. More data are also needed to determine if preoperative correction of iron-deficiency anemia will reduce the morbidity associated with anemia.

REFERENCES

1. Sim YE, Wee HE, Ang AL, et al. Prevalence of preoperative anemia, abnormal mean corpuscular volume and red cell distribution width among surgical patients in Singapore, and their influence on one year mortality. PLoS One 2017;12(8): e0182543.
2. Wu W-C, Schifftner TL, Henderson WG, et al. Preoperative hematocrit levels and postoperative outcomes in older patients undergoing noncardiac surgery. JAMA 2007;297(22):2481–8.
3. Hong FS, Sieradzki N, Pollock C, et al. Prevalence and causes of preoperative anaemia in elective major surgery patients. Intern Med J 2017;47(12):1400–4.
4. Abdullah HR, Sim YE, Hao Y, et al. Association between preoperative anaemia with length of hospital stay among patients undergoing primary total knee arthroplasty in Singapore: a single-centre retrospective study. BMJ Open 2017;7(6): e016403.

5. Sim YE, Sim S-ED, Seng C, et al. Preoperative anemia, functional outcomes, and quality of life after hip fracture surgery. J Am Geriatr Soc 2018;66(8):1524–31.

6. World Health Organization. Haemoglobin concentrations for the diagnosis of anaemia and assessment of severity. WHO/NMH/NHD/MNM/11.1. Available at: https://www.who.int/vmnis/indicators/haemoglobin.pdf. Accessed February 1, 2019.

7. Rosencher N, Kerkkamp HEM, Macheras G, et al. Orthopedic Surgery Transfusion Hemoglobin European Overview (OSTHEO) study: blood management in elective knee and hip arthroplasty in Europe. Transfusion 2003;43(4):459–69.

8. Gombotz H, Schreier G, Neubauer S, et al. Gender disparities in red blood cell transfusion in elective surgery: a post hoc multicentre cohort study. BMJ Open 2016;6(12):e012210.

9. Whitlock EL, Kim H, Auerbach AD. Harms associated with single unit perioperative transfusion: retrospective population based analysis. BMJ 2015;350:h3037.

10. Muñoz M, Acheson AG, Auerbach M, et al. International consensus statement on the peri-operative management of anaemia and iron deficiency. Anaesthesia 2017;72(2):233–47.

11. Busti F, Campostrini N, Martinelli N, et al. Iron deficiency in the elderly population, revisited in the hepcidin era. Front Pharmacol 2014;5:83.

12. Guralnik JM, Eisenstaedt RS, Ferrucci L, et al. Prevalence of anemia in persons 65 years and older in the United States: evidence for a high rate of unexplained anemia. Blood 2004;104(8):2263–8.

13. Muñoz M, Laso-Morales MJ, Gómez-Ramírez S, et al. Pre-operative haemoglobin levels and iron status in a large multicentre cohort of patients undergoing major elective surgery. Anaesthesia 2017;72(7):826–34.

14. Goodnough LT. Iron deficiency syndromes and iron-restricted erythropoiesis (CME). Transfusion 2012;52(7):1584–92.

15. Goodnough LT, Nemeth E, Ganz T. Detection, evaluation, and management of iron-restricted erythropoiesis. Blood 2010;116(23):4754–61.

16. Meynard D, Babitt JL, Lin HY. The liver: conductor of systemic iron balance. Blood 2014;123(2):168–76.

17. Ganz T. Systemic iron homeostasis. Physiol Rev 2013;93(4):1721–41.

18. Ganz T, Nemeth E. Iron sequestration and anemia of inflammation. Semin Hematol 2009;46(4):387–93.

19. Beattie WS, Karkouti K, Wijeysundera DN, et al. Risk associated with preoperative anemia in noncardiac surgery: a single-center cohort study. Anesthesiology 2009;110(3):574–81.

20. Karkouti K, Wijeysundera DN, Beattie WS, Reducing Bleeding in Cardiac Surgery (RBC) Investigators. Risk associated with preoperative anemia in cardiac surgery: a multicenter cohort study. Circulation 2008;117(4):478–84.

21. Saager L, Turan A, Reynolds LF, et al. The association between preoperative anemia and 30-day mortality and morbidity in noncardiac surgical patients. Anesth Analg 2013;117(4):909–15.

22. Abdullah HR, Sim YE, Sim YT, et al. Preoperative red cell distribution width and 30-day mortality in older patients undergoing non-cardiac surgery: a retrospective cohort observational study. Sci Rep 2018;8(1):6226.

23. Fowler AJ, Ahmad T, Phull MK, et al. Meta-analysis of the association between preoperative anaemia and mortality after surgery. Br J Surg 2015;102(11): 1314–24.

24. Chan DXH, Sim YE, Chan YH, et al. Development of the combined assessment of risk encountered in surgery (CARES) surgical risk calculator for prediction of

postsurgical mortality and need for intensive care unit admission risk: a single-center retrospective study. BMJ Open 2018;8(3):e019427.

25. Mueller MM, Van Remoortel H, Meybohm P, et al. Patient blood management: recommendations from the 2018 Frankfurt consensus conference. JAMA 2019; 321(10):983–97.

26. Chaves PHM, Xue Q-L, Guralnik JM, et al. What constitutes normal hemoglobin concentration in community-dwelling disabled older women? J Am Geriatr Soc 2004;52(11):1811–6.

27. Baron DM, Hochrieser H, Posch M, et al. Preoperative anaemia is associated with poor clinical outcome in non-cardiac surgery patients. Br J Anaesth 2014;113(3): 416–23.

28. Thein M, Ershler WB, Artz AS, et al. Diminished quality of life and physical function in community-dwelling elderly with anemia. Medicine 2009;88(2):107–14.

29. Cecchi F, Pancani S, Vannetti F, et al, Mugello Study Working Group. Hemoglobin concentration is associated with self-reported disability and reduced physical performance in a community dwelling population of nonagenarians: the Mugello Study. Intern Emerg Med 2017;12(8):1167–73.

30. Carabini LM, Zeeni C, Moreland NC, et al. Development and validation of a generalizable model for predicting major transfusion during spine fusion surgery. J Neurosurg Anesthesiol 2014;26(3):205–15.

31. Wu W-C, Smith TS, Henderson WG, et al. Operative blood loss, blood transfusion, and 30-day mortality in older patients after major noncardiac surgery. Ann Surg 2010;252(1):11–7.

32. Benjamin EJ, Virani SS, Callaway CW, et al. Heart disease and stroke statistics-2018 update: a report from the American Heart Association. Circulation 2018; 137(12):e67–492.

33. Isbister JP. The three-pillar matrix of patient blood management. ISBT Sci Ser 2015;10(S1):286–94.

34. Guinn NR, Guercio JR, Hopkins TJ, et al. How do we develop and implement a preoperative anemia clinic designed to improve perioperative outcomes and reduce cost? Transfusion 2016;56(2):297–303.

35. Perepu US, Leitch AM, Reddy S. Implementation of a preoperative anemia management clinic in a tertiary academic medical center. Blood 2016;128(22):1004.

36. Meybohm P, Goehring MH, Choorapoikayil S, et al. Feasibility and efficiency of a preoperative anaemia walk-in clinic: secondary data from a prospective observational trial. Br J Anaesth 2017;118(4):625–6.

37. Althoff FC, Neb H, Herrmann E, et al. Multimodal patient blood management program based on a three-pillar strategy: a systematic review and meta-analysis. Ann Surg 2018. https://doi.org/10.1097/SLA.0000000000003095.

38. Camaschella C. Iron-deficiency anemia. N Engl J Med 2015;373(5):485–6.

39. Ratcliffe LEK, Thomas W, Glen J, et al. Diagnosis and management of iron deficiency in CKD: a summary of the NICE guideline recommendations and their rationale. Am J Kidney Dis 2016;67(4):548–58.

40. Saxena S, Shulman IA, Johnson C. Effect of blood transfusion on serum iron and transferrin saturation. Arch Pathol Lab Med 1993;117(6):622–4.

41. Galesloot TE, Vermeulen SH, Geurts-Moespot AJ, et al. Serum hepcidin: reference ranges and biochemical correlates in the general population. Blood 2011; 117(25):e218–25.

42. Alleyne M, Horne MK, Miller JL. Individualized treatment for iron-deficiency anemia in adults. Am J Med 2008;121(11):943–8.

43. Ganzoni AM. Intravenous iron-dextran: therapeutic and experimental possibilities. Schweiz Med Wochenschr 1970;100(7):301–3.

44. Rimon E, Kagansky N, Kagansky M, et al. Are we giving too much iron? Low-dose iron therapy is effective in octogenarians. Am J Med 2005;118(10):1142–7.

45. Tolkien Z, Stecher L, Mander AP, et al. Ferrous sulfate supplementation causes significant gastrointestinal side-effects in adults: a systematic review and meta-analysis. PLoS One 2015;10(2):e0117383.

46. Cancelo-Hidalgo MJ, Castelo-Branco C, Palacios S, et al. Tolerability of different oral iron supplements: a systematic review. Curr Med Res Opin 2013;29(4): 291–303.

47. Clevenger B, Richards T. Pre-operative anaemia. Anaesthesia 2015;70(Suppl 1): 20–8, e6-e8.

48. Weiss G, Goodnough LT. Anemia of chronic disease. N Engl J Med 2005;352(10): 1011–23.

49. Goodnough LT, Skikne B, Brugnara C. Erythropoietin, iron, and erythropoiesis. Blood 2000;96(3):823–33.

50. Stein J, Dignass AU. Management of iron deficiency anemia in inflammatory bowel disease - a practical approach. Ann Gastroenterol Hepatol 2013;26(2): 104–13.

51. Dignass AU, Gasche C, Bettenworth D, et al. European consensus on the diagnosis and management of iron deficiency and anaemia in inflammatory bowel diseases. J Crohns Colitis 2015;9(3):211–22.

52. Kotkiewicz A, Donaldson K, Dye C, et al. Anemia and the need for intravenous iron infusion after Roux-en-Y gastric bypass. Clin Med Insights Blood Disord 2015;8:9–17.

53. Macdougall IC, Bircher AJ, Eckardt K-U, et al. Iron management in chronic kidney disease: conclusions from a "kidney disease: improving global outcomes" (KDIGO) controversies conference. Kidney Int 2016;89(1):28–39.

54. Macdougall IC, Bock AH, Carrera F, et al. FIND-CKD: a randomized trial of intravenous ferric carboxymaltose versus oral iron in patients with chronic kidney disease and iron deficiency anaemia. Nephrol Dial Transplant 2014;29(11):2075–84.

55. Onken JE, Bregman DB, Harrington RA, et al. A multicenter, randomized, active-controlled study to investigate the efficacy and safety of intravenous ferric carboxymaltose in patients with iron deficiency anemia. Transfusion 2014;54(2): 306–15.

56. Vadhan-Raj S, Strauss W, Ford D, et al. Efficacy and safety of IV ferumoxytol for adults with iron deficiency anemia previously unresponsive to or unable to tolerate oral iron. Am J Hematol 2014;89(1):7–12.

57. Auerbach M, Deloughery T. Single-dose intravenous iron for iron deficiency: a new paradigm. Hematol Am Soc Hematol Educ Program 2016;2016(1):57–66.

58. Chertow GM, Mason PD, Vaage-Nilsen O, et al. Update on adverse drug events associated with parenteral iron. Nephrol Dial Transplant 2006;21(2):378–82.

59. Kim Y-W, Bae J-M, Park Y-K, et al. Effect of intravenous ferric carboxymaltose on hemoglobin response among patients with acute isovolemic anemia following gastrectomy: the FAIRY randomized clinical trial. JAMA 2017;317(20):2097–104.

60. Blunden RW, Lloyd JV, Rudzki Z, et al. Changes in serum ferritin levels after intravenous iron. Ann Clin Biochem 1981;18(Pt 4):215–7.

61. Baird-Gunning J, Bromley J. Correcting iron deficiency. Aust Prescr 2016;39(6): 193–9.

62. Little DR. Ambulatory management of common forms of anemia. Am Fam Physician 1999;59(6):1598–604.

63. Zhao Y, Jiang C, Peng H, et al. The effectiveness and safety of preoperative use of erythropoietin in patients scheduled for total hip or knee arthroplasty: a systematic review and meta-analysis of randomized controlled trials. Medicine 2016; 95(27):e4122.

64. Grant MD, Piper M, Bohlius J, et al. Epoetin and darbepoetin for managing anemia in patients undergoing cancer treatment: comparative effectiveness update. Rockville (MD): Agency for Healthcare Research and Quality (US); 2013.

65. Devon KM, McLeod RS. Pre and peri-operative erythropoietin for reducing allogeneic blood transfusions in colorectal cancer surgery. Cochrane Database Syst Rev 2009;(1). CD007148. Available at: https://www.cochranelibrary.com/cdsr/doi/10.1002/14651858.CD007148.pub2/abstract.

66. Henke M, Laszig R, Rübe C, et al. Erythropoietin to treat head and neck cancer patients with anaemia undergoing radiotherapy: randomised, double-blind, placebo-controlled trial. Lancet 2003;362(9392):1255–60.

67. Leyland-Jones B, Semiglazov V, Pawlicki M, et al. Maintaining normal hemoglobin levels with epoetin alfa in mainly nonanemic patients with metastatic breast cancer receiving first-line chemotherapy: a survival study. J Clin Oncol 2005;23(25): 5960–72.

68. Rizzo JD, Brouwers M, Hurley P, et al. American Society of Hematology/American Society of Clinical Oncology clinical practice guideline update on the use of epoetin and darbepoetin in adult patients with cancer. Blood 2010;116(20): 4045–59.

69. Rizzo JD, Brouwers M, Hurley P, et al. American Society of Clinical Oncology/American Society of Hematology clinical practice guideline update on the use of epoetin and darbepoetin in adult patients with cancer. J Oncol Pract 2010; 6(6):317–20.

70. Muñoz M, Gómez-Ramírez S, Kozek-Langeneker S, et al. "Fit to fly": overcoming barriers to preoperative haemoglobin optimization in surgical patients. Br J Anaesth 2015;115(1):15–24.

71. Goodnough LT, Maniatis A, Earnshaw P, et al. Detection, evaluation, and management of preoperative anaemia in the elective orthopaedic surgical patient: NATA guidelines. Br J Anaesth 2011;106(1):13–22.

72. Peters F, Ellermann I, Steinbicker AU. Intravenous iron for treatment of anemia in the 3 perisurgical phases: a review and analysis of the current literature. Anesth Analg 2018;126(4):1268–82.

73. Froessler B, Palm P, Weber I, et al. The important role for intravenous iron in perioperative patient blood management in major abdominal surgery: a randomized controlled trial. Ann Surg 2016;264(1):41–6.

74. Na H-S, Shin S-Y, Hwang J-Y, et al. Effects of intravenous iron combined with low-dose recombinant human erythropoietin on transfusion requirements in iron-deficient patients undergoing bilateral total knee replacement arthroplasty. Transfusion 2011;51(1):118–24.

75. Bernabeu-Wittel M, Romero M, Ollero-Baturone M, et al. Ferric carboxymaltose with or without erythropoietin in anemic patients with hip fracture: a randomized clinical trial. Transfusion 2016;56(9):2199–211.

76. Keeler BD, Simpson JA, Ng O, et al. Randomized clinical trial of preoperative oral versus intravenous iron in anaemic patients with colorectal cancer. Br J Surg 2017;104(3):214–21.

77. Edwards TJ, Noble EJ, Durran A, et al. Randomized clinical trial of preoperative intravenous iron sucrose to reduce blood transfusion in anaemic patients after colorectal cancer surgery. Br J Surg 2009;96(10):1122–8.

78. Khalafallah AA, Yan C, Al-Badri R, et al. Intravenous ferric carboxymaltose versus standard care in the management of postoperative anaemia: a prospective, open-label, randomised controlled trial. Lancet Haematol 2016;3(9): e415–25.

79. Jin L, Kapadia TY, Von Gehr A. Feasibility of a preoperative anemia protocol in a large integrated health care system. Perm J 2019;23 [pii:17-200]. Available at: http://www.thepermanentejournal.org/issues/2019/winter/6975-feasibility-of-a-preoperative-anemia-protocol-in-a-large-integrated-health-care-system.html.

80. Bosch X, Montori E, Guerra-García M, et al. A comprehensive evaluation of the gastrointestinal tract in iron-deficiency anemia with predefined hemoglobin below 9mg/dL: a prospective cohort study. Dig Liver Dis 2017;49(4):417–26.

81. Goodnough LT, Schrier SL. Evaluation and management of anemia in the elderly. Am J Hematol 2014;89(1):88–96.

82. Coban E, Timuragaoglu A, Meriç M. Iron deficiency anemia in the elderly: prevalence and endoscopic evaluation of the gastrointestinal tract in outpatients. Acta Haematol 2003;110(1):25–8.

83. van Zeben D, Bieger R, van Wermeskerken RK, et al. Evaluation of microcytosis using serum ferritin and red blood cell distribution width. Eur J Haematol 1990; 44(2):106–9.

84. Pascual-Figal DA, Bonaque JC, Manzano-Fernández S, et al. Red blood cell distribution width predicts new-onset anemia in heart failure patients. Int J Cardiol 2012;160(3):196–200.

85. Van Craenenbroeck EM, Conraads VM, Greenlaw N, et al. The effect of intravenous ferric carboxymaltose on red cell distribution width: a subanalysis of the FAIR-HF study. Eur J Heart Fail 2013;15(7):756–62.

86. Anaemia Management in Chronic Kidney Disease: Partial Update 2015. Section 4: Diagnostic evaluation and assessment of anaemia. NICE Guideline, No. 8. National Clinical Guideline Centre (UK). London: Royal College of Physicians (UK); 2015.

87. den Elzen WPJ, de Craen AJM, Wiegerinck ET, et al. Plasma hepcidin levels and anemia in old age. The Leiden 85-Plus Study. Haematologica 2013;98(3):448–54.

88. Wittkamp C, Traeger L, Ellermann I, et al. Hepcidin as a potential predictor for preoperative anemia treatment with intravenous iron: a retrospective pilot study. PLoS One 2018;13(8):e0201153.

89. Skikne BS. Serum transferrin receptor. Am J Hematol 2008;83(11):872–5.

90. Drakou A, Margeli A, Theodorakopoulou S, et al. Assessment of serum bioactive hepcidin-25, soluble transferrin receptor and their ratio in predialysis patients: correlation with the response to intravenous ferric carboxymaltose. Blood Cells Mol Dis 2016;59:100–5.

91. Katsanos K, Cavalier E, Ferrante M, et al. Intravenous iron therapy restores functional iron deficiency induced by infliximab. J Crohns Colitis 2007;1(2):97–105.

92. Soppi ET. Iron deficiency without anemia: a clinical challenge. Clin Case Rep 2018;6(6):1082–6.

93. Lopez A, Cacoub P, Macdougall IC, et al. Iron deficiency anaemia. Lancet 2016; 387(10021):907–16.

94. Ponikowski P, Voors AA, Anker SD, et al. 2016 ESC guidelines for the diagnosis and treatment of acute and chronic heart failure: the task force for the diagnosis and treatment of acute and chronic heart failure of the European Society of Cardiology (ESC)Developed with the special contribution of the Heart Failure Association (HFA) of the ESC. Eur Heart J 2016;37(27):2129–200.

95. Ponikowski P, van Veldhuisen DJ, Comin-Colet J, et al. Beneficial effects of long-term intravenous iron therapy with ferric carboxymaltose in patients with

symptomatic heart failure and iron deficiency†. Eur Heart J 2015;36(11): 657–68.

96. Anker SD, Comin Colet J, Filippatos G, et al. Ferric carboxymaltose in patients with heart failure and iron deficiency. N Engl J Med 2009;361(25):2436–48.

Moving?

Make sure your subscription moves with you!

To notify us of your new address, find your **Clinics Account Number** (located on your mailing label above your name), and contact customer service at:

Email: journalscustomerservice-usa@elsevier.com

800-654-2452 (subscribers in the U.S. & Canada)
314-447-8871 (subscribers outside of the U.S. & Canada)

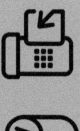

Fax number: 314-447-8029

Elsevier Health Sciences Division
Subscription Customer Service
3251 Riverport Lane
Maryland Heights, MO 63043

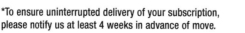

Printed and bound by CPI Group (UK) Ltd, Croydon, CR0 4YY

03/10/2024

01040406-0013